Contents

Contents

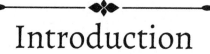

Introduction

Welcome, dear readers, to a thrilling journey!

This book, "Project Well-Being: Embracing Digital Technology in Care," promises to be your steadfast companion as you venture into the vibrant world of digital tech within care settings.

Are you ready to transform the lives of the people you support? Shattering the invisible barriers that have kept them from the exhilarating digital world? Do you imagine a future where everyone, irrespective of age or health, can join the global digital community? If your heart is echoing a resounding "yes," then you've chosen the perfect guide.

We understand that diving into the digital domain can feel a bit like stepping onto an alien planet, especially for those accustomed to more traditional care settings. But worry not! Just as Neil Armstrong took one small step and leaped into history, you too will find your footing in this new landscape, guided by our practical, easy-to-follow steps and tips.

In Project Well-Being, we endeavour to make the seemingly complex world of digital technology not just approachable, but downright enjoyable! Our aim is to help you and the individuals you care for benefit from the myriad opportunities that digital tech has to offer – from touch screen tables that can trigger precious memories for people living with dementia, to music therapy that can soothe the soul and stimulate the brain, to app-based solutions that open up endless possibilities for learning and entertainment.

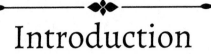

Introduction

Throughout the chapters of this book, you'll discover how to prepare for the arrival of digital tech in your care setting, how to introduce these technologies to the people you support, and how to effectively manage and optimise their use over time.

We'll also delve into how to navigate the challenges that come with change, ensuring you feel empowered and confident in your digital journey.

By the end of this book, your care setting will be on the path to becoming a digitally inclusive environment, where everyone can experience the joy and benefits of the digital world.

You'll have the knowledge and tools to enrich lives, stimulate minds, and bring smiles to faces, all through the power of digital tech.

So, let's embark on this exciting journey together! Embrace the spirit of discovery, of learning, and of creating a more inclusive digital future for all. Welcome to Project Well-Being!

Part I: Preparation for Digital Technology in Care Settings

Chapter 1: Preparing for Your Interactive Table Arrival.

Welcome aboard the Tiny Tablet train! This first stop on your journey to digital inclusion in care settings is all about preparation.

In this chapter, we'll share the best practices and essential steps to take before your Tiny Tablet arrives, eliminating as much "trial and error" as possible, and setting you on a sure path to success.

Our program is not merely about introducing a piece of technology; it's about creating an engaging, stimulating environment that caters to the physical, cognitive, and emotional needs of the people you support.

We want to equip you with the knowledge and confidence to enjoy touch screen technology with your people from day one, creating memorable moments and meaningful interactions.

Before your Tiny Tablet arrives, there are a few important tasks to complete:

1. Setting Up a Google Account:

To ensure you can hit the ground running with downloading apps and activities, you'll need to set up a Google account. Visit www.google.com, tap "sign in" at the top right, and follow the prompts to create a new account. It's a simple process that opens the door to a world of digital possibilities.

Chapter 1: Preparing for Your Interactive Table Arrival.

2. Preparing for Social Media Engagement:

On the day of delivery, you'll want to share the excitement with families of the people you support and the wider community. Prepare some content for your social media platforms to post on the big day. Remember to tag us on Facebook, Instagram, TikTok, Twitter, Pinterest & LinkedIn—we love to share in your joy and progress!

Now, let's talk about the Tiny Tablets themselves. The primary difference between our Fixed Height and Variable Height tablets is the electronic motor that allows the latter to adjust to different heights.

This feature makes the Variable Height table an excellent choice for individuals in specialty wheelchairs, those unable to leave their bed, or for facilitating group activities. However, for safety, if the Variable Height table encounters any resistance while adjusting, it will automatically stop to prevent accidents.

Chapter 1: Preparing for Your Interactive Table Arrival.

3. Gathering Personal Reference Points:

For people who have cognitive impairment or communication difficulties, engaging with them effectively often requires personalised stimuli.

Contact their families to obtain a list of personal reference points. These might include favourite places, holidays, previous addresses, important life events, favourite singers, songs, movies, TV shows, hobbies, sports teams, or memorable sports events.

You can use Google Earth, YouTube, Wikipedia, or Chrome to research these reference points, turning them into a treasure trove of engagement opportunities. Alternatively, consider using our "My Story So Far" PDF, which families can fill out, providing a wonderful snapshot of each persons life.

Remember, each step of preparation is a stride towards creating a vibrant, inclusive digital environment. So let's roll up our sleeves and get ready for an exciting journey with Tiny Tablets in your care setting!

Chapter 2: Managing the Day of Delivery

Hooray! The big day has arrived.

Your Tiny Tablet is here, and it's time to usher in a new era of digital engagement in your care setting.

As you unwrap your tablet with our delivery team, we promise the experience will be as exhilarating as unwrapping a much-anticipated holiday gift. But instead of a fleeting moment of joy, this gift promises to deliver enduring engagement, stimulation, and joy to your individuals.

First things first, ensure that your Tiny Tablet is fully charged. Plug it in and press the button at the back of the tablet to bring it to life.

As it hums into action, you can almost sense the anticipation in the air! After a brief loading time, your Tiny Tablet will be ready for action, its screen glowing with potential.

Chapter 2: Managing the Day of Delivery

The display panel at the back of the tablet will show the battery percentage.

It might dim after a while, but a quick tap will bring it back to light.

If you opted for a Variable Height table, you'll find the button to adjust the screen's height conveniently located at the back as well.

Next up, let's get your Tiny Tablet connected. Dive into the settings to link up with your Wi-Fi.

If there are any firewalls to tackle, enlist the assistance of your IT department. They'll help ensure your new device is smoothly integrated into the network.

And don't forget about the Bluetooth connection! You can pair up Bluetooth devices through the same settings menu. For example, Bluetooth Speakers for enhanced sound, Bluetooth Headphones for private viewing/audio books/listening to music and other SEN devices.

Chapter 2: Managing the Day of Delivery

While you're in the settings, don't miss the screenshot function.

It's a nifty feature found 5 icons from the bottom. Make sure it's ticked to enable the screenshot ability.

This function allows you to capture whatever is on the screen at that time, effectively 'freezing the moment.' You can then revisit these moments in the "Gallery" app, a wonderful tool for reflecting on engagement activities and progress.

So, are you ready to turn on, tune in, and venture forth into the exciting world of digital engagement?

With your Tiny Tablet ready and raring to go, you're all set to transform the lives of the people you support through the magic of digital technology.

Welcome to the future of care!

Chapter 3: Ensuring Your Setup is Ready to Go

Congratulations! You're now at the thrilling stage of setting up your Tiny Tablet.

This chapter will guide you through the steps to get your digital powerhouse up, running, and filled with exciting apps that will captivate the individuals you care for.

Firstly, log into the Play Store using the Google account details you established for your care setting.

With access to thousands of apps, the Play Store is your gateway to a world of interactive possibilities. Now it's time to start downloading apps.

But where to start, you might wonder? Don't worry, we've got you covered! We've included a list of the most popular apps used in care settings (which are all free to download) near the back of this guide to help you get started.

Plus, your Tiny Tablet comes with a few pre-installed apps to spark immediate engagement.

Chapter 3: Ensuring Your Setup is Ready to Go

Consider downloading the suite of Google apps that are incredibly beneficial for you and the individuals you care for.

Apps like Google Drive, Gmail, Chrome, Google Meet, and Google Earth offer a myriad of ways to engage, learn, and connect.

For easy access, group these apps into a folder. Just hold your finger on an app icon and drag it over another app. Voila! You've created a folder that you can name and easily locate.

Do remember, though, not all apps are created equal. Some are developed specifically for phones and might not look as good or function as well on a large screen.

If you come across an app that doesn't quite hit the mark, don't fret. Just delete it and find a similar one that works better. The beauty of the Play Store is its vastness—with new apps being developed and uploaded every week, you're sure to find the perfect fit.

To delete an app, simply hold your finger on the app icon and drag it to the left of the screen towards the bin. Agree to uninstall, and you're all set.

So, take a deep breath and dive into the exciting world of apps, exploring, experimenting, and discovering the best ways to enrich the lives of the people you support through digital technology. With each app you download, you're opening a new door to engagement, stimulation, and joy. Let's get those apps rolling!

Chapter 4: Exploring the Free Software Available

Welcome to Chapter 4, where we dive into the treasure trove of free software available on the Google Play Store.

Free apps are a fantastic way to explore the vast array of possibilities without breaking the bank. But remember, as the saying goes, there's no such thing as a free lunch.

These apps may display ads during use. But fear not, we've got two fantastic solutions to keep those pesky pop-ups at bay:

1. **Stay offline when you can:** Keep your Wi-Fi turned off when it's not required. This stops ads from making unsolicited appearances during your digital adventures. Accessing your Wi-Fi and Bluetooth settings is as easy as swiping down on your screen at the top left to bring up a quick menu.
2. **Employ ad-blocking software:** We recommend AdGuard, a free and user-friendly tool for ad blocking. Simply download it from the Play Store, follow the steps to allow it to block ads, and switch it on when prompted. With AdGuard in your corner, you can enjoy an ad-free experience!

Once your Tiny Tablet is set up and ad-free, it's time to organise your apps. Put your sensory apps into a named folder for easy access. Some brilliant sensory apps to kickstart your collection include Magic Fluids, Fireworks, Baby Bubble, Sensory Fish, Galaxy Particles, and My Reef 3D. Also, make sure Google Earth and YouTube are downloaded and that you're connected to your Wi-Fi.

Chapter 4: Exploring the Free Software Available

Before you introduce the tablet to those you care for, get to know it yourself.

Experiment with the different apps and functions. Familiarity breeds confidence, and confidence is infectious!

Start your digital journey with your more relaxed people in your care (if there are more than one). Remember, it's natural for some to voice concerns like, "I've lived for... years without using something like that, why do I need to start now?" It's a valid point.

This new, sizeable piece of technology can seem intimidating. But with your enthusiasm and guidance, they'll soon see the fun and engagement it can bring.

We recommend practicing switching between apps and using the Tiny Tablet's functions with your team. This will make the transition much smoother when you're ready to introduce it to those you care for.

Most importantly, don't put pressure on yourself, and have fun! Remember, this is a journey of discovery for everyone involved.

And don't forget, we're here to help! If you have any questions or need additional support, feel free to email us at info@inspired-inspirations.com, and we'll call you back to assist. So, are you ready to dive into the vibrant world of free software? Let's go!

Part II: Familiarising People You Support with Digital Tech

Chapter 5: Strategies for Approaching the People you Support

Welcome to Chapter 5, where we discuss the heart of our mission: effectively introducing the Tiny Tablet to the individuals you care for.

New technology can feel a bit like a new language, and it's our job to translate it in a way that feels comfortable, exciting, and accessible.

One way to introduce the Tiny Tablet is to make a lively entrance into the common area. Fire up some tunes on YouTube, and let the music do the talking. Dance, sing, and encourage the people you support to join in. This approach breaks the ice and introduces the Tiny Tablet as a source of joy and fun!

An alternative approach is to opt for a more intimate setting. Gather a few people in a room and explore the apps together, starting with the sensory ones. This more personalised method allows individuals to familiarise themselves with the technology in a less crowded environment.

Chapter 5: Strategies for Approaching the People you Support

One strategy that has seen great success is the 1-2-1 activities approach.

Picture this: you and someone you care for, comfortably settled in the living room, exploring a sequence of engaging activities. The trick is to introduce digital tech through intrigue, entice them into touching the screen through sensory apps.

Start with the mesmerising Magic Fluids, move on to the delightful Baby Bubbles, then feed the fish in the enchanting My Reef 3D. Next, take a trip down memory lane with Google Earth, visiting their old home. Cap it off with a song from their favourite singer on YouTube and a group word search.

This approach offers a balance of individual attention and group involvement.

You'll often find that as the more relaxed people you support start enjoying the activities, the typically less-engaged people grow curious and join the fun.

Remember, there is no one-size-fits-all approach. Find the method that resonates best with those you support and staff. And above all else, keep it fun and lighthearted. The goal is to make this new technology feel like a friendly and familiar part of their day.

So let's dive in and create some wonderful digital experiences together!

Chapter 6: Introducing Tech Tools to People Living with Dementia

Welcome to Chapter 6, where we will dive into how to successfully introduce the Tiny Tablet to people living with dementia. While the journey may have its challenges, remember that the rewards of connection, joy, and mental stimulation make the effort worthwhile.

1. **Ease into the experience:** Begin by introducing one app at a time. This allows the person to explore, learn, and become comfortable with each function before moving onto the next. Patience is key here; remember that less is more when it comes to processing new information.
2. **Familiarity is your friend:** Choosing apps that the people you support for can relate to can make the experience less daunting. This could mean puzzles they've always loved, games they've played before, or music that sparks joy and memories. The familiarity can help minimise any feelings of frustration or confusion.
3. **Size matters:** A simple yet effective strategy is to increase the font size on the tablet. This can greatly enhance readability for individuals who may have vision difficulties.
4. **Visual cues to the rescue:** Adding visual cues or reminders about what the tablet is for can greatly reduce confusion. This could be a note, a sticker, or even a familiar image.
5. **Provide guided support:** Encourage and guide them through each app and function. Your support will be invaluable in making this a positive experience for them.
6. **Simplicity is king:** Keep the tablet's interface simple and straightforward. Avoid apps that are overly complicated or challenging to navigate.

Chapter 6: Introducing Tech Tools to People Living with Dementia

Bringing technology into the lives of people living with dementia may not always be straightforward, but it's an endeavour filled with promise and potential. The benefits of this process are profound, offering not just engagement, but rich, meaningful interaction that can greatly enhance the quality of life for the people you care for.

The journey to familiarise them with the Tiny Tablet may take time, but remember, every moment spent is an investment in their well-being. It's an opportunity to weave digital threads into the tapestry of their daily activities, adding vibrancy, variety, and a wealth of cognitive stimulation.

Guiding the people you support through this process requires patience, understanding, and a gentle touch. However, it also calls for creativity! Each person is unique, with their own history, preferences, and pace of learning. By customising the experience to their needs and interests, you can help them uncover the joy and sense of accomplishment that comes with mastering new skills.

The Tiny Tablet can be more than just an innovative tool; it can become a catalyst for connection. It offers a portal to their past, a platform for their present, and a gateway to new experiences. It's a medium through which they can express themselves, engage with others, and explore the world around them.

Chapter 7: Enriching the Lives of People Living with Dementia via Touch Screen Tech

The use of touch screen technology, such as the Tiny Tablet, opens up a new horizon of possibilities for enriching the lives of individuals living with dementia. This chapter explores the numerous ways this innovative tool can aid in cognitive improvement, offer engaging activities, and generally enhance the quality of life for dementia patients.

- **Music and Memory:**

There's a profound connection between music and memory that persists even when dementia has eroded other cognitive abilities.

Music has the ability to evoke strong emotions and recall memories deeply embedded within an persons consciousness. Studies suggest that people living with dementia can often remember melodies long after faces, names, and words have faded.

Music can thus be a powerful tool to boost mood, reduce agitation, and improve focus. The Tiny Tablet allows people to access a vast library of songs, tunes, and melodies, creating their personal playlists of familiar tracks. This immersion in music can have a positive impact on their quality of life, reducing anxiety and depression, and enhancing their overall well-being.

Chapter 7: Enriching the Lives of People Living with Dementia via Touch Screen Tech

- **Cognitive Stimulation and Learning:**

The touch screen technology of the Tiny Tablet encourages interactivity, which can stimulate cognitive functioning and improve memory. It offers games and puzzles tailored to the cognitive abilities and personal interests of the people you support. The process of learning to navigate the tablet itself can also be an engaging activity that stimulates cognitive function.

- **Physical Engagement:**

The Tiny Tablet can also be used to promote physical activity, which is beneficial for overall health and well-being. Simple games that require individuals to use their fingers to interact with the touch screen can encourage fine motor skills and coordination.

- **Sensory Enrichment:**

The tablet's interactive nature and brightly coloured screen can stimulate visual senses. For those with sensory impairment, the tablet can be adjusted to suit their comfort level, ensuring an engaging experience.

Chapter 7: Enriching the Lives of People Living with Dementia via Touch Screen Tech

- **Managing "Sundowning":**

Touch screen activity tables can be a useful tool in managing sundowning, a common symptom of dementia, characterised by increased confusion and agitation during the late afternoon and evening. Engaging activities on the touch screen can serve as a distraction, reducing the intensity of sundowning symptoms. It provides a safe and controlled environment for activity, reducing the risk of accidents.

Our initial encounter with "sundowning" was with a charming lady who, each day at 3 pm, felt compelled to leave the care home, believing she had dinner to prepare. Her increasing restlessness was a daily concern.

To divert her from her afternoon agitation, we introduced her to a group engaging in a word search. However, when she hinted at needing to leave, we promptly asked about where she got married. We found the church on Google Earth, presenting it to her as she turned to leave.

Her face lit up at the sight, launching her into a captivating account of her wedding day. This joyful reminiscing demonstrated the potential of technology in fostering engagement and distraction from behaviour of concern.

Chapter 7: Enriching the Lives of People Living with Dementia via Touch Screen Tech

Here are several more strategies that could help to distract and reduce sundowning symptoms:

1. **Music Therapy**: Encourage the person you support to listen to their favourite songs or participate in a sing-along. Music has been shown to have a calming effect and can stimulate happy memories.
2. **Physical Activity**: Arrange for some light exercise such as, chair aerobics, or simple stretching exercises. Physical activity can help to reduce restlessness and agitation.
3. **Art and Crafts**: Activities like digital drawing, digital cross stitch, or other crafts can keep hands busy and minds focused, reducing the agitation that can lead to sundowning.
4. **Mind-Stimulating Games**: Games that stimulate the mind such as puzzles, word searches, Sudoku, or memory games can be a great way to keep residents engaged and distracted.
5. **Relaxation Techniques**: Breathing exercises, meditation, or gentle yoga can help to calm the mind and body.
6. **Storytelling or Reading**: Encourage people you support to share their stories or read to them from their favourite books. This can offer a comforting distraction and a sense of connection.

Remember, every person is unique and what works for one person may not work for another. It may take some experimentation to find out what activities are most effective for each person you support.

Chapter 7: Enriching the Lives of People Living with Dementia via Touch Screen Tech

- **Combating Dehydration:**

Forgetting to stay hydrated is a common issue among individuals with dementia. Touch screen activity tables can help combat this issue by integrating hydration reminders into interactive games and activities, promoting regular water intake.

- **Reducing Reliance on Anti-psychotic Drugs:**

Emerging research suggests that engaging activities on touch screen tables can help reduce the reliance on anti-psychotic drugs commonly used to manage dementia symptoms. These activities provide a positive and engaging distraction, reducing anxiety and stress levels, and thereby decreasing the need for medication.

- **Virtual Exploration and Reminiscence:**

Google Earth, when used on a touch screen activity table, can be a wonderful tool for reminiscence therapy. It allows individuals to revisit places that hold significant memories, stimulating positive emotions and social interaction. It enables individuals to virtually revisit their childhood homes, wedding venues, former workplaces, and favourite holiday destinations. Don't worry if you evoke emotions, this is a great sign and can be managed through music and media.

Chapter 8: Enhancing Recovery for Stroke Patients with Digital Tech

Memory, Learning & Cognitive Improvement

A stroke can have a profound impact, not just physically, but cognitively as well, often affecting memory and learning capabilities. This can be challenging for survivors who seek to regain their independence and confidence post-stroke. Digital technology can be designed to address this issue, fostering the revival of positive memories and promoting learning.

Digital technology's primary cognitive advantage lies in its potential to boost a patient's memory and learning skills. Apps designed for memory games and cognitive training stimulate the brain and improve recall, while educational apps foster the acquisition of new skills and knowledge.

Regular usage of these apps can help stroke survivors enhance their cognitive functions and regain self-confidence.
In addition, Tiny Tablets empower stroke survivors by giving them control over their recovery process. The sense of accomplishment experienced through completing app-based tasks or achieving set goals can bring immense satisfaction.

For memory and learning enhancement, apps such as Lumosity, Elevate, and MyBrainTrainer offer a wide array of games, puzzles, and personalised cognitive training programs. These tools can play a pivotal role in enriching the lives of stroke survivors, enhancing cognitive abilities, and fostering a sense of independence.

Chapter 8: Enhancing Recovery for Stroke Patients with Sensory Impairment Digital Tech

Stroke can often result in sensory impairments such as loss of sight or hearing, which can significantly hinder a person's ability to communicate and interact. Tiny Tablets can help alleviate these challenges by providing an intuitive and accessible communication platform.

One of the significant advantages of Tiny Tablets is that they enable effective communication despite sensory loss. The touch screen technology provides an easy-to-understand interaction method, reducing the frustrations associated with traditional communication means.

Moreover, numerous apps cater explicitly to sensory impairments, thus providing a more inclusive experience.

Apps like Be My Eyes, Ava, and MagnusCards can enhance sensory experiences for stroke survivors. They provide visual assistance, real-time captions for the hearing-impaired, and step-by-step guidance for daily tasks, respectively, making them more accessible for those with sensory impairments.

Thus, Tiny Tablets not only ease communication frustrations but also improve the overall quality of life and reduce feelings of isolation.

Chapter 8: Enhancing Recovery for Stroke Patients with Digital Tech

Interactivity

Physical and cognitive challenges post-stroke often lead to social isolation and reduced ability to interact with others. However, Tiny Tablets can play a significant role in improving these aspects of recovery by promoting interactivity and social engagement.

Tiny Tablets offer a plethora of interactive activities, ranging from games and puzzles to educational resources and rehabilitation exercises. Engaging with these activities can contribute to physical and cognitive improvement, thereby aiding the rehabilitation process. Furthermore, the social interaction features offered by the Tiny Tablets, such as video calls and access to social media platforms, can help combat feelings of loneliness and isolation. They also provide a platform for stroke survivors to connect with online communities and support groups, fostering shared experiences and emotional support.

Exercise

Exercise, physiotherapy, and stretching are critical components of stroke rehabilitation. They help restore physical abilities, improve confidence, and thereby, enhance the overall quality of life. Tiny Tablets enable stroke survivors to participate in activities promoting movement and stretching, leading to improved rehabilitation outcomes.

Apps such as Lumosity and YouTube offer cognitive and physical exercises, and easy-to-follow videos for gentle exercises like chair yoga and seated aerobics, respectively. By using these apps, stroke survivors can improve their physical abilities and regain confidence in their bodies.

Chapter 8: Enhancing Recovery for Stroke Patients with Digital Tech

Relaxation

High stress and anxiety levels are common among stroke survivors, which can hamper their recovery process.

Relaxation techniques such as meditation and mindfulness can help alleviate stress and promote deep, restorative sleep, essential for physical and mental recovery. Tiny Tablets can aid this process by offering various apps that foster relaxation and mindfulness.

Apps like Calm and Headspace provide guided meditations, breathing exercises, and sleep stories, all designed to reduce stress and promote relaxation and mental clarity. These apps are particularly beneficial for stroke survivors who may have mobility limitations or difficulties accessing traditional relaxation methods.

The inclusion of relaxation and mindfulness in stroke rehabilitation can positively influence overall health. Stress reduction can help lower blood pressure and improve cardiovascular health, while quality sleep can aid in physical and mental recovery.

Therefore, by utilising the relaxation and mindfulness apps available on Tiny Tablets, stroke survivors can significantly enhance their recovery process.

Chapter 8: Enhancing Recovery for Stroke Patients with Digital Tech

Music & Media

Music and media play a significant role in aiding stroke survivors' recovery process. Interestingly, research indicates that stroke survivors often retain their memory for music, even when other memory forms are impaired. Music can uplift mood, reduce agitation, and improve focus, all beneficial for the recovery process.

A Tiny Tablet Touch Screen Activity Table can serve as a valuable tool for integrating music and media into stroke rehabilitation. Easy access to a range of music and media apps, such as Spotify and YouTube, can provide a wide variety of musical genres and artists, thus allowing patients to find music that helps them relax and focus.

Personalised playlists can also be created for patients, enhancing their engagement and enjoyment during rehabilitation. Further, the Tiny Tablet can provide access to educational videos or podcasts, helping stroke survivors stay informed about their condition and strategies for managing their symptoms, thereby providing mental stimulation during their rehabilitation sessions.

In conclusion, incorporating music and media into stroke rehabilitation can significantly enhance recovery outcomes. Using a Tiny Tablet Touch Screen Activity Table, stroke survivors can access a wide range of resources, which can improve their overall well-being, mood, and focus. By personalising their rehabilitation process, stroke survivors can regain control of their lives, fostering a sense of empowerment and independence.

Part III: Progression of Technology Implementation

Chapter 9: Days 2-7: Establishing a Digital Rhythm

Okay, let's dive into the second part of our digital adventure - a week of fine-tuning, personalising, and getting jiggy with our Tiny Tablet!

Here's a day-to-day breakdown of how to get into the groove and make your Tiny Tablet feel like home for every person in your care.

Day 2: Getting Organised

Our digital housekeeping day. Start by setting up app folders for each type of app, making it easier to find. It's like spring cleaning for your Tablet - only less dust and more fun! To set up specific folders for apps, press your finger on the chosen app icon and drag it over a similar app - bingo, you have a folder. Then give it a name, e.g. Sensory Apps

And, remember, duplicating app icons is not just okay; it's encouraged! There's no limit on digital real estate here.

Day 3: Personalise Away!

Time to make each persons experience uniquely theirs. Use the "My Story So Far" fact finding PDF (available for download in our online resource hub) to collect information about each resident. This will help tailor their experience.

Our Care Manager Top Tip for the day? Set up folders for each person you support containing their favourite apps. That way, any staff member can quickly identify which apps each person enjoys most.

Chapter 9: Days 2-7: Establishing a Digital Rhythm

Day 4: Screenshots for the Win!

It's time to get snappy with the Screenshot function. It's perfect for recording any activity completed and tracking scores or times taken. To take a screenshot, simply click the camera icon in the toolbar, and voila! The picture is stored in your gallery app under "screenshots." Easy-peasy lemon squeezy, right? You can then email these records or store them in digital care plans or even Google Drive to share with families. Picture perfect.

Day 5: Let's Get Physical!

No, we're not going to break into an Olivia Newton-John song (though we could, thanks to our Tiny Tablet). Instead, we're adding a sprinkle of physical exercise to our digital stew.

Each morning, you can find an exercise video on YouTube designed for our dear older friends. Care settings using their tablets for physical exercise (in addition to mental stimulation) have seen an overall increase in well-being of the people who are being supported. There are also care-specific physical exercise training programs available, currently being used on thousands of Tiny Tablets.

Chapter 9: Days 2-7: Establishing a Digital Rhythm

Day 6: Planning Ahead

Our Care Manager Top Tip today? Start working on a daily activity plan. Don't worry; it's just a guide, not a strict timetable. This plan can help keep things organised and ensure every person you support gets the most out of their Tiny Tablet time.

Day 7: Flexibility is Key!

Remember, the daily activity plan is merely a suggestion, not a commandment. Feel free to adapt it, tweak it, or throw it out of the window if it doesn't suit your individuals. After all, every day in a care setting is a little different, and that's the beauty of it.

So, that's our rhythm for the first week. By now, the Tiny Tablet should feel like a familiar friend for both staff and supported people. So, keep exploring, keep personalising, and, most importantly, keep having fun!

Chapter 10: Days 8-14: Broadening the Scope of Digital Usage

Great job, everyone! We're moving onto week two with our trusty Tiny Tablet sidekick. Now that we've familiarised ourselves with the basics, it's time to delve deeper and bring some therapeutic fun into the mix. Yes, we're talking about reminiscence therapy. It's time to turn those digital pixels into portals to the past.

Now that we have a week under our belts, let's take a moment to reflect. Are our app folders working? Are the personalised folders for each individual helpful? What apps are proving popular? This is our digital pit-stop, where we tweak, assess, and fine-tune to make the rest of the journey even smoother.

Day 8: Opening the Gates of Reminiscence

Let's kick off with creating our 'Memory Lane' folder right on the home screen. This little vault of nostalgia can hold apps tailored specifically for reminiscence therapy - think photo album apps, YouTube channels streaming classic TV shows, movies, you name it.

Now that our folder is set, let's fill it with goodies. Use apps like Google Photos or the in-built Gallery to navigate through pictures from the past. Feel free to gab about the moments, people, places in these photos. The goal here is to foster a sense of connectedness, promote social interactions and just have a good time strolling down memory lane.

Chapter 10: Days 8-14: Broadening the Scope of Digital Usage

Day 9: Check Out Other Apps & DIY Digital Scrapbooks

Yes, there are plenty of apps out there, and it's high time we explore them! Just like the vast universe, the app world is filled with endless possibilities. From new games to educational content, cooking recipes, and brain teasers, there's something for everyone.

Get ready to wear your creative hats! We're crafting digital scrapbooks and journals using apps like Canva or Google Docs. These are the canvases for your resident artists to paint their past - add photos, captions, memories, and anything that sparks joy.

Day 10: Trial and Error Day

We know it sounds a tad scary, but this day is all about embracing the unexpected. Download new apps, try out different settings, and see what clicks. Remember, there are no mistakes, just unexpected adventures.

Let's share our digital wins! What apps are working well? Any fun stories to share? Remember, the Tiny Tablet experience is a team effort, so don't shy away from sharing your tips and tricks.

Chapter 10: Days 8-14: Broadening the Scope of Digital Usage

Day 11: Energise with Exercise

Exercise isn't just great for physical health; it's a mood-booster and a cognitive kickstarter. Let's blend in some physical activity into our digital routine - chair exercises, yoga, or even impromptu dance parties using YouTube videos or live stream one of the many interactive exercise classes designed for those in care settings. Pick whatever fits your individuals' physical abilities and get the party started.

Day 12: Document and Discover

Remember the screenshot function we learned about? Time to put it into action. Document activities and progress of the people you support. Not only does it help track engagement, but it also serves as a great tool to identify areas that could use a little improvement.

Today, we're also doing our backups. While it might sound dull compared to discovering new apps, it's crucial for safeguarding our hard work. Think of it as protecting your digital treasure.

Day 13: Personalisation Station

Here's a fun exercise - grab the "My Story So Far" PDF and get to know your people even better. This wonderful tool can be used to understand your everyones" interests, hobbies, and past experiences.

Use this information to personalise their Tiny Tablet experience, and watch as their faces light up with delight!

Chapter 10: Days 8-14: Broadening the Scope of Digital Usage

Day 14: Toast to Two Weeks

Two weeks in, and look how far we've come! Let's celebrate with a trip down 'Memory Lane'. A viewing party of classic TV shows or a shared digital scrapbook session, perhaps? You decide!

And there you have it. Our journey through Week 2 with the Tiny Tablet is all about reminiscing the past, creating joy in the present, and shaping a brighter future.

Let's keep the fun rolling!

Chapter 11: Days 15-21: Solidifying the Digital Learning Experience

Well, we've got two fantastic weeks behind us and now it's time to make our relationship with Tiny Tablet as solid as a rock.

Week 3 is all about getting artsy, challenging the brain, socialising, exploring, and finding calm. Ready to dive in? Let's go.

Day 15: The Picasso Day

We're all artists deep down, and today we'll bring that out with the Drawing Desk app. From pencils to spray paint, this app is the digital art studio we've been waiting for. Import images to trace or use as a reference, and let the creative juices flow!

Day 16: Writer's Paradise

For those who've got a way with words, we've got the Memo app. Jot down notes, reminders or maybe a haiku or two on a virtual sticky note. And guess what? These can be set to pop up as reminders on specific dates and times. Cool, huh?

Care Manager Top Tip: Try incorporating the artwork or notes into an individuals room decor. It's like having a personalised piece of art!

Day 17: Sudoku Time

Ready to put those grey cells to work? Let's take on some Sudoku puzzles! With apps tailored to different difficulty levels, we have challenges for every Sudoku samurai out there.

Chapter 11: Days 15-21: Solidifying the Digital Learning Experience

Day 18: Bingo Bonanza

Bingo time with Bingo Bash app! Small group or large, the app's got us covered with various themes and patterns. Bingo, anyone?

Day 19: Virtual Adventure

On day 19, we're globe-trotting with the Google Arts & Culture app. Art, history, virtual museum tours - it's a whirlwind cultural adventure, right from our comfy armchairs!

Day 20: Quiz and Chill

QuizUp app, anyone? From history buffs to pop-culture fans, we have quizzes for everyone. People can compete against each other or even take on other players online. Game on!

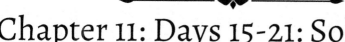

Chapter 11: Days 15-21: Solidifying the Digital Learning Experience

Day 21: Digital Skill-Up

The final day of week three is all about learning something new. With the Udemy app, we can dive into topics from cooking and crafting to tech and business. It's like having a personal tutor in your pocket!

Throughout the week, we've got a few other tricks up our sleeve:

- Fancy a laugh? Check out the TikTok app for short, hilarious videos that are guaranteed to bring a smile to everyone's faces.

- To help keep everyone in touch with loved ones, we'll be using the Skype and Zoom apps for voice, video calls and messages. Let's fight loneliness and isolation together!

- The Calm app offers guided meditations and soothing sounds to help us unwind and relax.

- And for a grand finale, we'll be using the Heads Up app for an energetic game of charades and the Tiny Beans app for sharing memories and photos with loved ones.

Chapter 12: Celebrating the Completion of Your First 3 Weeks

Whoop, whoop! Three cheers for the tablet troopers.

You've just completed three full weeks of navigating through the digital universe on your Tiny Tablet(s), hand-in-hand with the people you support. Isn't it amazing how the time flew by?

By now, you might have noticed that some of people you support are more engaged, others are more communicative, and a few even seem to be having a cracking good time!

Isn't it something when Mrs. Jones starts telling stories about her childhood during the reminiscence tours or when Mr. Smith finally nails that Sudoku puzzle he's been grappling with? It's moments like these that make our digital adventure so rewarding.

Now, don't for a minute think we're leaving you stranded in this new digital landscape. Nope, we're just a booking away! To continue your journey and confront any pesky obstacles you might be facing, we strongly recommend scheduling an online training session with us.

Visit www.inspired-inspirations.com to find out how.

Chapter 12: Celebrating the Completion of Your First 3 Weeks

When staff embrace touchscreen technology and engage the people they support, the transformation is nothing short of magical.

People who were previously disengaged may suddenly perk up, quieter folks may start chattering away, and don't be surprised if a common interest in '50s pop music or French cuisine mends old feuds in the care setting.

So, get your party hats on, do a little victory dance, and bask in the glow of your achievement. The past three weeks were just the beginning, and we can't wait to see where this journey takes us next.

Remember, we're here for you every step of the way, so please feel free to reach out if you need any more help or guidance. After all, every good adventure is better with friends!

Here's to more exploration, more learning, and more fun. Onwards and upwards, digital trailblazers!

Chapter 13: Examples of Effective Weekly Plans

"Plans are nothing; planning is everything." Who knew old Dwight D. Eisenhower's wisdom would be just as applicable to our digital adventure as to his wartime strategy?

Now that you've had your first few weeks of exploration with your Tiny Tablet(s), it's time to create a rhythm, a routine, a... drumroll, please... weekly plan!

But don't panic! We're not asking you to draft a battle strategy. We're just talking about a simple schedule to add some structure and predictability to the digital fun we're having. As the saying goes, 'variety is the spice of life', and this is especially true when it comes to planning activities for the people you support. It also provides structure and excitement for what's to come.

So, we've put together a few examples of weekly plans that have worked wonderfully in other care settings.

Tiny Tablet Table Exercise & Movement Planner

TIME	MONDAY	TUESDAY	WEDNESDAY	THURSDAY	FRIDAY	SATURDAY	SUNDAY
Early AM	Cycling tour (using pedals) group or individual activity	Seated exercises via YouTube or Apps	Hand exercises via YouTube or Apps – ideal for those from bed	Full body exercises via YouTube or Apps	Seated exercises via YouTube or Apps	Breathing exercises via YouTube or Apps	Yoga for the elderly
Mid AM	Hand/foot massages to aid blood flow along to music.	Fun App based games while standing.	Piano Morning (perfect Piano, Learn to Play section)	Hand/foot massages to aid blood flow along to music.	Free hand drawing apps, writing names, letters and numbers	App based mobility exercise to improve movement and stretching. Jigsaws & Painting by Numbers	Reaction based app games, winner stays on EG Air Hockey
Early PM	App based mobility exercise to improve movement and stretching. Jigsaws & Painting by Numbers	Reaction based app games, winner stays on EG Air Hockey	App based mobility exercise to improve movement and stretching. Jigsaws & Painting by Numbers	Reaction based app games, winner stays on EG Air Hockey	Fun App based games while standing.	Word searches	Hand/foot massages to aid blood flow along to music.
Evening	Painting by Numbers evening with calming music	Dance Night, with a play list put together by residents	Free hand drawing apps, writing names, letters and numbers	Painting by Numbers evening with calming music	Upbeat Dance Night, with a play list put together by residents	Classical Dance Night, with a play list put together by residents	Piano evening (perfect Piano, Learn to Play section)
Night Time	Any activities to calm or relax restless residents, or those who cant sleep, in particular breathing exercise and focussed deep breathing.						

Chapter 13: Examples of Effective Weekly Plans

Tiny Tablet Table Planner
Residential Care

TIME	MONDAY	TUESDAY	WEDNESDAY	THURSDAY	FRIDAY	SATURDAY	SUNDAY
Early AM	Cycling tour (using pedals) group or individual activity	Seated exercises via YouTube or Apps	Hand exercises via YouTube or Apps – ideal for those from bed	Full body exercises via YouTube or Apps	Seated exercises via YouTube or Apps	Breathing exercises via YouTube or Apps	Yoga for the elderly
Mid AM	Sensory room visits. Sensory activities for those who can't leave their rooms	Bedroom visits and 121 activities with those unable or not wanting to leave their rooms	Story time, listening to an audio book, Audible	Group reminiscence afternoon on Google Earth. Where did you work? Share & discuss	Quiz Morning, Who Wants to be a Millionaire, Trivial Pursuit.	Bedroom visits and 121 activities with those unable or not wanting to leave their rooms	Live Streaming Religious Services
Early PM	Bingo	Group reminiscence afternoon on Google Earth. Holiday locations & discuss	Creativity afternoon, painting by numbers, pottery app	Competition time, air hockey/ 4 in a row/ bowling championship	Group reminiscence afternoon on Google Earth. Where did you grow up? Share & discuss	Replay historic sport events. Favourite boxing/football/rugby/ tennis/cricket etc, highlights to play and	Streaming previous days sports at request
Evening	Comedy Night with comedians from the past	Movie night	Bedroom visits and 121 activities with those unable or not wanting to leave their rooms	Music evening, learn to play a new song via Perfect Piano	Casino night, Roulette apps etc	Sing – a – longs and dancing evening	Relaxation evening, Soothing Sounds and picture
Night Time	Any activities to calm or relax restless residents, or those who cant sleep, great for 121 time and story telling too.						
Additional activities to include	Video calling, personal learning/interests, 121 living room time, managing any challenging behaviour that may arise, board games, brain and memory training etc etc						

Tiny Tablet Table Planner for those with mid–later stages of Dementia

TIME	MONDAY	TUESDAY	WEDNESDAY	THURSDAY	FRIDAY	SATURDAY	SUNDAY
Early AM	Sensory room visits. Sensory activities for those who can't leave their rooms	Hand massage along to Nature Sounds App	Breathing exercises via YouTube or Apps	Sensory room visits. Sensory activities for those who can't leave their rooms	Hand exercise via YouTube or Apps	Breathing exercises via YouTube or Apps	Hand massage along to Nature Sounds App
Mid AM	Music Therapy, watch and listen to favourite singers from the past	Sensory room visits. Sensory activities for those who can't leave their rooms	Music Therapy, watch and listen to favourite singers from the past	Story time, listen to an audio book	Quiz Morning/My House of Memories/ Memory games	Sensory room visits. Sensory activities for those who can't leave their rooms	Live Streaming Religious Services
Early PM	Seasonal Streaming (live stream bird feeders, zoos, spring watch etc)	Group reminiscence afternoon on Google Earth. Visit familiar places	Sensory room visits. Sensory activities for those who can't leave their rooms	Creativity, free drawing, painting by numbers.	Group reminiscence afternoon on Google Earth. Visit familiar places	Replay historic sport events. Favourite boxing/football/rugby/ tennis/cricket etc, highlights	Music Therapy, watch and listen to favourite singers from the past
Evening	Movie night with classic clips from the past	Musical evening on the instrument apps, piano, drums, xylophone etc	Bedroom visits and 121 activities with those unable or not wanting to leave their rooms	Musical evening on the instrument apps, piano, drums, xylophone etc	Comedy Night with comedians from the past	Music Therapy, watch and listen to favourite singers from the past	Relaxation evening, Soothing Sounds and pictures
Night Time	Any activities to calm or relax restless residents, or those who cant sleep, great for 121 time and story telling too.						
Additional activities to include	Video calling, personal learning/interests, 121 living room time, managing any challenging behaviour that may arise, board games, brain and memory training etc etc						

Chapter 13: Examples of Effective Weekly Plans

Tiny Tablet Table Planner Quizzes & Brain Training

TIME	MONDAY	TUESDAY	WEDNESDAY	THURSDAY	FRIDAY	SATURDAY	SUNDAY
Early AM	Maths Duel app 1v1 winner stays on	Train your brain: Memory	Train your brain: Visioupatial	Train your brain: Coordination	Who wants to be a Millionaire	Train your brain: Language	Suduko
Mid AM	Who wants to be a Millionaire	Math, group maths quiz	Maths Duel app 1v1 winner stays on	My House of Memories	Train your brain: Reasoning	Wheel of Fortune	Pastimes 14 in 1 or 2 Player Pastimes
Early PM	Train your brain: Attention	Scrabble	History Quiz: various apps	Scrabble	Maths Duel app 1v1 winner stays on. End of week winner!	Who wants to be a Millionaire	Various Board Games
Evening	Word Search by Wixot	Various Board Games	Word with Friends	Water Sort	Various Board Games	Jeopardy group game	My House of Memories
Night Time	Any activities to calm or relax restless residents, or those who cant sleep, great for 121 time and story telling too.						

Tiny Tablet Table Planner Sheltered Scheme

TIME	MONDAY	TUESDAY	WEDNESDAY	THURSDAY	FRIDAY	SATURDAY	SUNDAY
Early AM	Cycling tour (using pedals) group or individual activity	Seated exercises via YouTube or Apps	Hand exercises via YouTube or Apps – ideal for those from bed	Full body exercises via YouTube or Apps	Seated exercises via YouTube or Apps	Breathing exercises via YouTube or Apps	Yoga for the elderly
Mid AM	Maths Morning – Maths Duel and Math apps	Music Quiz and fun, name that year	Story time, listening to an audio book, Audible	Group reminiscence afternoon on Google Earth. Where did you work? Share & discuss	Quiz Morning, Who Wants to be a Millionaire, Trivial Pursuit.	Free time fun	Live Streaming Religious Services
Early PM	Bingo	Group reminiscence afternoon on Google Earth. Holiday locations & discuss	Creativity afternoon, painting by numbers, pottery app	Competition time, air hockey/ 4 in a row/ bowling championship	Free time fun	Replay historic sport events. Favourite boxing/football/rugby/tennis/cricket etc, highlights to play.	Streaming previous days sports at request
Evening	Comedy Night with comedians from the past	Movie night	Music, watch and listen to favourite singers from the past	Music evening, learn to play a new song via Perfect Piano	Casino night, Roulette apps etc	Sing – a – longs and dancing evening	Relaxation evening, Soothing Sounds and picture
Additional activities to include	Video calling, personal learning/interests, 121 living room time, digital crafts, board games, brain and memory training, learning languages, Digital skills training etc etc						

Chapter 13: Examples of Effective Weekly Plans

You'll notice a few things about these plans:

1. **Variety:** Each day of the week has a mix of activities - from physical exercises and reminiscence therapy to artistic adventures and trivia challenges.
2. **Consistency:** While the activities vary, the schedule remains somewhat consistent. This gives the people you support something to look forward to each day.
3. **Personal Touch:** The plans are tailored to suit the interests and abilities of the people you support. Remember, the Tiny Tablet(s) should be a source of joy, not stress.
4. **Flexibility:** The plan isn't rigid. If a session of virtual globe-trotting sparks a conversation about travel, let the conversation flow. If a Sudoku puzzle is proving too tough, switch to a lighthearted game of digital charades.

Remember, these are just examples. Feel free to get creative and come up with a plan that best suits your residents.

After all, you're the maestro conducting this digital symphony! Just keep it balanced, keep it fun, and everything else will fall into place.

Happy planning, tablet maestros!

Part IV: Maximising Digital Technology Utilisation

Chapter 14: Fostering Cross-Generational Communication

"When I was your age, we didn't even have the internet!"

Does that sound familiar?

Well, it's time to change the tune. With the Tiny Tablet in your care setting, we're here to bridge the generational gap and foster some fun cross-generational communication. Because who says tech is only for the young?

From the people you support sharing stories from their youth, to their grandchildren explaining the latest internet memes, there's a world of knowledge and laughter to be shared across the ages. And guess what? The Tiny Tablet can be your very own digital bridge!

Let's Explore!

1. Tiny Tablet Tutors: Next time a young visitor stops by, why not invite them to join a Tiny Tablet activity? Your people might just amaze them with their digital prowess, and the little ones will love helping out!

2. Game on, Generation Z! Is there a better way to bond than over a game? No matter if it's Bingo, Sudoku, or perhaps even a virtual tour of the Louvre, the Tiny Tablet is ready for all ages.

3. Memory Lane: Grandparents taking grandchildren on a virtual tour of places they've visited using Google Earth? Now, that's what we call time travel! With storytelling, learning, and bonding rolled into one, it's the perfect activity to keep everyone engaged and create special moments.

Chapter 14: Fostering Cross-Generational Communication

Teamwork Makes the Dream Work

Your youngest staff members are an invaluable asset when it comes to Tiny Tablet use. With their digital confidence and eagerness, they can help those you care for complete the "My Life So Far" fact-finding document, creating stronger bonds in the process.

This document, which which there is a copy in Chapter 21, is designed to help newly supported people settle in, providing staff with a unique insight into their life experiences and interests.

Apps like YouTube, Google Earth, Wikipedia and Chrome can be used to take people to reference points, deepening the conversation and making it even more meaningful.

Care Manager Top Tip

Get family members involved in filling out the "My Life So Far" document. They could share anecdotes and details that you may otherwise miss, fostering stronger communication between the care team and family members.

So there you have it! Embrace the joy of learning and sharing across generations, all powered by your Tiny Tablet. After all, the digital wave is for everyone to ride!

Chapter 15: Facilitating Late-in-Life Learning

Let's banish the saying, "You can't teach an old dog new tricks," shall we?

It's high time we embraced the joy and benefits of lifelong learning. Remember, it's never too late to pick up a new hobby, learn a new skill, or even a new language!

Whether the people you support are budding Beethovens or aspiring polyglots, there's a wealth of knowledge at their fingertips - all thanks to the Tiny Tablet.

Here's how you can help keep their brains buzzing with new information.

New Skills, New Thrills!

1. ¡Hola! Bonjour! 你好!: Did you know that learning a new language is great for cognitive agility? With the Babbel app on the Tiny Tablet, your service users can pick up Spanish, French, Chinese, and many more languages! Now that's a conversation starter!

2. Tickling the Ivories: Maybe it's been a lifelong dream to play 'Moonlight Sonata' on the piano. With the Perfect Piano app, your individuals can learn to play songs and melodies in a fun, interactive way. Who knows, you might have the next Mozart in your midst!

3. Curiosity Corner: Encourage your people to dive deep into their interests. Whether it's birdwatching, the history of railroads, or even quantum physics, the Tiny Tablet can be used to research these topics. And why stop there? Invite them to prepare mini presentations on their chosen topics to share with their peers.

Chapter 15: Facilitating Late-in-Life Learning

Breaking Down Barriers

Using new technology can be daunting for some. To ease any hesitations and build confidence, we have the Digital Inclusion guide available in our online hub.

This comprehensive guide walks through every step of using the Tiny Tablet, from unboxing to downloading apps.

Care Manager Top Tip

Pair up people based on shared interests or skills they'd like to learn. This buddy system can help create a supportive learning environment where they can help each other and celebrate their progress together.

So, get set to tap into the power of late-in-life learning with the Tiny Tablet. After all, every day is a school day, no matter your age!

Chapter 16: Crafting Engaging Playlists

Ah, the power of a good playlist! It can bring back memories, uplift spirits, energise workouts, or even provide a soothing backdrop for relaxation. And with the Tiny Tablet, curating the perfect playlist for your individuals is as simple as tap, tap, tap!

Whether it's a nostalgic tune from their youth, a classical symphony to accompany an afternoon nap, or a foot-tapping number for a mini dance party, playlists can be a versatile tool in your activity repertoire. Here's how you can fine-tune the playlist creation process:

Platform Proficiency

1. Spotify Savvy: From blues to Bach, and jazz to jive, Spotify is a musical cornucopia where you'll find every possible genre, artist, and song. Create a profile for your care setting and craft custom playlists for different moods, events, or even individual people you care for. Music therapy session? There's a playlist for that. Sunday brunch? There's a playlist for that too!

2. YouTube Virtuoso: YouTube is not just about cute cats and funny fails. It's a treasure trove of music videos, historical clips, sports events, and much more. It's perfect for creating visual playlists that can serve as a talking point and stimulate reminiscence.

Chapter 16: Crafting Engaging Playlists

Personalisation Power

1. Family Input: Encourage families to join the playlist creation process. They can create a Spotify playlist with their loved one's favourite songs, childhood memories, or even tunes that marked special events in their lives. It's a beautiful way to maintain connections and personalise their music experience.
2. Person-Specific Playlists: Dive deep into each persons interests, past, and preferences. A playlist with songs from someones wedding? Or tunes from their hometown? The possibilities are endless, and so are the chances for personalised engagement.

Care Manager Top Tip

Commit a bit of time initially to understand the nuances of the Tiny Tablet, Spotify, YouTube, and the unique musical tastes of people you support. Set up folders and playlists in such a way that any team member can easily navigate and use them.

This will ensure that even those who are slightly technophobic can confidently utilise the Tiny Tablet to its full potential.

Remember, music is a universal language, and with the Tiny Tablet, you have an orchestra at your fingertips! So, let the music play and the good times roll.

Chapter 17: Harnessing the Most Popular Activities for Optimal Engagement

Let's dive right into the magic of engagement and explore some of the most effective and fun ways to use the Tiny Tablet in your care setting.

Virtual Visits: The Power of Video Calling

Welcome to the new age of communication where physical distance is no longer a barrier. Say hello to video calls, a virtual window to their loved ones, and a fantastic tool to facilitate much-needed face-to-face interactions. We're living in a digital world where staying in touch is just a click away.

The first step towards harnessing the power of video calls is to familiarise yourself with some of the most popular video calling apps.

The Tiny Tablet is compatible with an array of platforms such as Zoom, Skype, Google Duo, Facebook Messenger, and WhatsApp. Each of these platforms has its own set of unique features, but they all serve the same purpose: to make communication simpler, more engaging, and more personal.

Zoom, for instance, offers high-quality video and audio and can host multiple participants at once, making it perfect for family gatherings or social events. Skype and Google Duo are other reliable options, each boasting user-friendly interfaces that even the most technologically timid can master. Facebook Messenger and WhatsApp, on the other hand, are more than just video calling apps. They're multifunctional platforms where users can send text messages, share photos, and even participate in group chats.

Chapter 17: Harnessing the Most Popular Activities for Optimal Engagement

Video calls can help make people feel more connected to their loved ones, enhancing their overall well-being. It's a wonderful sight to see a persons face light up when they see their grandchildren's antics or when they have a heart-to-heart with their old friends. Video calls can capture these precious moments.

But the power of video calling extends beyond merely social connections. In today's world, video calls are playing an increasingly crucial role in healthcare. Telemedicine is the way of the future, offering patients access to healthcare professionals without leaving the comfort of their residence. For the people you support, this means no stressful commutes, no long waiting room times, and less exposure to potential health risks. Instead, they can schedule virtual appointments with their healthcare providers, right from the Tiny Tablet.

It's not just traditional medical consultations that can benefit from video calling technology. Physical therapy, psychiatric consultations, and even wellness check-ins can be conducted virtually. With video calling, people can have their needs addressed promptly, comfortably, and effectively.

Video calling is a potent tool in your hands, capable of enhancing lives in several ways. It brings their loved ones closer, reduces feelings of loneliness, offers access to healthcare, and ultimately, adds a sparkle to their everyday life. So go ahead, bring the world to those in your care with the power of video calling.

Chapter 17: Harnessing the Most Popular Activities for Optimal Engagement

The World at Their Fingertips: Reminiscence Tours on Google Earth and Beyond

Imagine if you could offer the people you support a round-the-world trip, a chance to explore the breathtaking Pyramids of Egypt, the stunning canals of Venice, or the mesmerising cherry blossoms of Japan—all from the comfort of their own rooms. Sound like a dream?

With Google Earth, this dream becomes a reality. With just a few swipes on their Tiny Tablet, your people can traverse the globe, rekindle old memories, and even create some new ones along the way.

Google Earth is more than just a geographical tool—it's a virtual time machine.

People can revisit the street they grew up on, gaze at the house where they raised their family, or walk down memory lane, passing by their old school or favourite park.

All those memories hidden under the cobwebs of time can be dusted off, creating an opportunity for those you care for to share their stories, sparking meaningful conversations, and connecting with others.

Chapter 17: Harnessing the Most Popular Activities for Optimal Engagement

This wonderful tool can also provide a safe passage for people to revisit their favourite holiday spots. Did they ever share their love for the sandy beaches of Hawaii or the rustic charm of an old European city? Now, they can take a virtual stroll, feeling the sand between their toes or hearing the distant church bells toll, stirring up the memories of the beautiful times they spent there.

The magic of Google Earth doesn't stop there. This technology allows people to go on a virtual tour of places they always wanted to visit but never got the chance. Perhaps someone you support always dreamt of visiting the Eiffel Tower or exploring the mysteries of the Great Wall of China. Now, they can do it all while enjoying a cup of tea in their favourite armchair.

To add an extra layer of fun and engagement, consider organising themed reminiscence afternoons.

During these special events, people can take turns playing the tour guide, leading their peers through the streets of their chosen destinations, sharing anecdotes, experiences, and stories. Whether it's the nostalgia-filled lanes of their hometown or the stunning vistas of a foreign country, each tour will be a unique journey, full of discovery and shared experiences.

Chapter 17: Harnessing the Most Popular Activities for Optimal Engagement

Now, let's take it a step further with the power of a web browser like Google Chrome.

Imagine the potential of "Then and Now" explorations, comparing historical images of a location with its contemporary appearance. Using Chrome, you can pull up old photographs, news stories, or articles about a place, then switch back to Google Earth to see how it has changed over the years.

People you support can see how their childhood home or school has transformed, compare the bustling cityscapes or tranquil countrysides of yesteryears with their modern counterparts. The juxtaposition of the old and the new can stimulate vivid recollections, evoke deep emotions, and provide a rich context for discussion and sharing.

Incorporating Google Earth and Chrome in your care setting can thus not only help in engaging people in a fun, interactive manner but also stimulate their cognitive functions and contribute to their overall well-being. So, embark on this exciting journey, and let the people you support hold the world in their hands!

Chapter 17: Harnessing the Most Popular Activities for Optimal Engagement

Exploring Linguistic Horizons: Language Tutorials on YouTube and Beyond

Language learning can be an enriching and exciting experience at any age, and the benefits it provides are not merely limited to acquiring a new skill. It helps sharpen the mind, improves memory and concentration, boosts confidence, and fosters cultural understanding.

With the power of platforms like YouTube and language learning apps like Babbel, people you support can tap into this fountain of cognitive benefits while adding a fun, engaging element to their daily routine.

YouTube is a veritable treasure trove of language learning resources, offering a plethora of tutorials and lessons that cater to learners at all levels. From the comfort of their Tiny Tablet, people can immerse themselves in basic conversation practice, dive deep into the nuances of grammar, or build their vocabulary across a range of topics.

These YouTube tutorials are delivered in an engaging, interactive format, making language learning fun and less intimidating. With the ability to pause, rewind, and replay the lessons, people can learn at their own pace, reducing the pressure and increasing the joy of learning.

Chapter 17: Harnessing the Most Popular Activities for Optimal Engagement

But the power of technology in language learning doesn't stop at YouTube. Applications like Babbel offer a more structured and comprehensive approach to learning a new language or brushing up on one already learnt.

Babbel's lessons are designed by a team of language experts, linguists, and teachers, and are tailored to the learner's native language, ensuring an effective and personalised learning experience.

With Babbel, people can dive into the intricacies of languages like Spanish, French, Italian, German, and many more, with lessons spanning various aspects of language learning, including listening, reading, writing, and speaking. The app also includes review sessions to reinforce what's been learnt and a speech recognition feature to help perfect pronunciation.

Language learning isn't just about the cognitive benefits; it also has a significant social aspect. For people who come from different countries or have families who speak different languages, learning a new language or honing their skills in a known language can foster a greater sense of connection. It can make them feel closer to their cultural roots, improve communication with their loved ones, and foster a sense of belonging.

Chapter 17: Harnessing the Most Popular Activities for Optimal Engagement

Moreover, language learning can be a communal activity.

Consider organising language learning groups where people can practice speaking with each other, share what they've learnt, and even teach others. It's a great way to stimulate social interaction, collaboration, and mutual support among those who are being supported.

So, equip the people you support with the power of language learning through YouTube and apps like Babbel.

Turn on the tablet, tune in to a lesson, and watch as the world of words unfolds before them, breaking barriers, fostering connections, and bringing joy and enrichment to their everyday lives.

Chapter 17: Harnessing the Most Popular Activities for Optimal Engagement

The Joy of Discovery: Exploring the World with Wikipedia

Dive headfirst into the endless ocean of information that is Wikipedia.

It's an incredible platform that unlocks a universe of knowledge, ranging from historical events to scientific discoveries, cultural nuances to technological advancements. With just a few taps on their Tiny Tablet, people can access a treasure trove of knowledge, catered to their individual interests, curiosity, and pace.

Wikipedia provides an opportunity for people to recall the past, learn something new, satisfy their curiosity, or simply enjoy the thrill of exploring an endless array of topics. Have they ever wondered about the architectural styles of the Renaissance? Are they interested in the life and works of a particular author or artist? Do they want to understand more about the cosmos, the animal kingdom, or the digital world?

Wikipedia is their gateway to all these worlds and more.

What's more, Wikipedia isn't just about reading. It's an interactive platform that encourages users to delve deeper into topics of interest.

With an extensive network of hyperlinks, a single topic can lead to the discovery of numerous related topics, leading users on an exciting journey of interconnected knowledge. This aspect can stimulate cognitive functions and nurture a habit of lifelong learning.

Chapter 17: Harnessing the Most Popular Activities for Optimal Engagement

Another feature of Wikipedia that can be particularly enjoyable for people is the availability of numerous historical articles. People can reminisce about major events that took place in their lifetime, explore historical contexts, and understand how the world has changed over the years. It's like having a personal time machine at their fingertips!

But while Wikipedia is an excellent resource, it's crucial to bear in mind that it is a collaborative platform that can be edited by anyone.

Therefore, it's good practice to verify the information found on Wikipedia with other reputable sources, especially when exploring complex or contentious topics.

Encouraging people you support to check the references listed in Wikipedia articles can be a useful way to ensure they're getting reliable information, fostering critical thinking and information literacy.

It's also worth noting that Wikipedia isn't just available in English; it's multilingual. People who are native speakers of other languages or are learning new languages can access Wikipedia in numerous languages, making it an excellent resource for language learning and maintenance.

Chapter 17: Harnessing the Most Popular Activities for Optimal Engagement

In addition, Wikipedia isn't just about text.

Many articles come with images, diagrams, maps, and even sound clips that can enrich the learning experience. The platform is continuously evolving, with new articles and updates being added every day, ensuring there's always something new to discover.

In a nutshell, Wikipedia offers a world of exploration, discovery, and learning, making it a powerful tool for fostering engagement, intellectual stimulation, and joy in the journey of lifelong learning. So, empower the people you support with the thrill of discovery; equip them with their Tiny Tablet, guide them to Wikipedia, and let the joy of learning light up their days.

Chapter 17: Harnessing the Most Popular Activities for Optimal Engagement

Expanding Horizons: Embracing the Internet with Google Chrome

Foster digital inclusion in your care setting with the power of Google Chrome, a user-friendly web browser designed to provide a seamless internet experience. With Chrome, you're essentially giving your individuals a key to a limitless world of knowledge, entertainment, and exploration - right at their fingertips.

Exploring the internet opens up numerous possibilities for the people you support. They can delve into their interests, research their questions, explore new hobbies, or simply enjoy browsing through pictures and videos. With Google Chrome, the internet is like an interactive library, constantly updated and infinitely diverse.

Chrome's versatility enables those you care for to make the most of their online time. They can look up pictures, search for specific websites, watch videos, and use it as a reference point for discussions or activities. Whether they're interested in gardening, history, music, travel, or any other topic, they can find a wealth of resources online.

But Chrome isn't just about individual exploration. It can also be used to enhance group activities and discussions. For instance, you can search for and display images related to a discussion topic, watch documentaries or instructional videos together, or take virtual tours of museums, zoos, or other places of interest.

Chapter 17: Harnessing the Most Popular Activities for Optimal Engagement

What's more, Google Chrome takes news consumption to a new level.

Instead of passively watching television news, those you support can actively engage with the news online. With a simple search, they can access articles, videos, podcasts, and interactive content from multiple sources. This not only provides a more comprehensive understanding of the news but also allows people to explore the news topics that interest them most. They can follow live updates, delve into background information, read different perspectives, and even interact with the news through comments and social sharing.

Google Chrome also makes it easy to customise the browsing experience to meet the needs and preferences of each individual. With features like bookmarks and history, people can easily save and revisit their favourite websites. The browser's settings can be adjusted to increase font size, change screen brightness, or enable voice search for easier navigation.

Additionally, Chrome comes with a built-in translation feature, making it an excellent tool for language learning or for people who are more comfortable reading in a language other than English. They can navigate websites in their preferred language, further enhancing their browsing experience.

So, let's gear up to unlock the full potential of the internet for your people. Empower them with Google Chrome, guide them through its features, and watch as they experience the joy of discovery, learning, and engagement that the internet offers. It's time to redefine what internet browsing can mean for those you support.

Chapter 17: Harnessing the Most Popular Activities for Optimal Engagement

A Symphony of Senses: Exploring the World of Sensory Apps

One of the most compelling features of the Tiny Tablet is its ability to bring a sensory world to life through a variety of sensory apps. These apps are more than just interactive tools; they're doorways to experiences that can engage the senses, soothe the mind, and inspire a sense of wonder.

With bright visuals, soothing sounds, and engaging interactions, sensory apps can create a peaceful and calming environment, perfect for reducing anxiety.

From mesmerising colour patterns to relaxing ambient sounds, these apps are designed to bring tranquility and happiness. This can be particularly beneficial for people who may be dealing with stress, restlessness, or difficulty focusing.

On the other hand, sensory apps aren't only about calmness and relaxation; they can also be exciting and fun, stimulating curiosity and joy. They offer a wide range of activities, from creating dazzling light shows to making music with virtual instruments. With such a variety, there's a sensory app to fit any mood, interest, or need.

Chapter 17: Harnessing the Most Popular Activities for Optimal Engagement

Moreover, sensory apps promote social interaction. Many of these apps support "multi-touch," meaning that multiple users can interact with the app at the same time. This opens up opportunities for shared experiences and collaborative play, helping people connect with each other in enjoyable and meaningful ways.

Imagine a group of those you care for creating a beautiful piece of digital art together, or a pair working as a team to solve a musical puzzle.

But the magic of sensory apps doesn't stop there. For people with sensory impairments, these apps can provide stimulation and engagement in a manner few other resources can.

For example, for those with visual impairments, certain apps offer heightened audio feedback. Similarly, people with hearing difficulties can immerse themselves in visually rich and vibrant applications.

Furthermore, sensory apps can also bring the advantages of a sensory room directly to those people who may have difficulty accessing them. With the Tiny Tablet, the multi-sensory experiences can travel wherever they're needed, offering the joy and benefits of sensory stimulation to all residents, regardless of mobility.

Chapter 17: Harnessing the Most Popular Activities for Optimal Engagement

Lastly, sensory apps can support cognitive function.

The interactive nature of these apps can help improve motor skills, focus, and memory. They encourage active engagement, require decision-making, and reward curiosity, all of which contribute to cognitive health.

Sensory apps are not just games or tools; they're an innovative approach to promoting well-being, stimulating the senses, and bringing joy to the day of those you care for.

So why not dive into the world of sensory apps and experience the rich tapestry of sensations they have to offer? With the Tiny Tablet, a world of sensory stimulation is literally at your fingertips.

Chapter 17: Harnessing the Most Popular Activities for Optimal Engagement

Mind Gym: Tapping into the Potential of Cognitive Stimulation Apps

Ready to turn your care setting into a cognitive workout zone? Thanks to a plethora of brain-training games and apps designed to challenge the mind, stimulating cognitive function while entertaining those you support has never been easier.

But let's not stop there. Adding a dash of friendly competition with a leaderboard and a weekly prize can transform this cognitive exercise into a thrilling brain Olympics!

With cognitive stimulation apps, the Tiny Tablet transforms into a personal brain trainer, offering a myriad of puzzles, challenges, and games to stretch the mind. These exercises target different areas of cognition, such as memory, attention, problem-solving, and processing speed.

From classic games like chess and Sudoku to innovative apps that adapt to individual skill levels, there's something to cater to everyones' preference and cognitive fitness level.

Cognitive stimulation isn't a one-size-fits-all kind of thing, and the beauty of these apps lies in their variety. There are memory games that help people keep their recall sharp, pattern recognition games to challenge their logic, and even language games to support verbal fluency and comprehension. By providing a diversity of games, you'll ensure that everyone gets a well-rounded cognitive workout and stays engaged.

Chapter 17: Harnessing the Most Popular Activities for Optimal Engagement

Now, let's talk about taking it up a notch with a dose of competition.

After all, a little friendly rivalry can make cognitive exercise more exciting! By setting up a leaderboard, you'll foster a sense of community among the people you support as they cheer each other on and vie for the top spot. What's more, a weekly prize could serve as a tangible motivation, encouraging everyone to participate and do their best.

And that's not all. Tracking progress is also a vital part of this cognitive stimulation journey. By keeping track of peoples' scores, you'll gain valuable insights into their cognitive health over time. The screenshots of the scores can be stored in each persons' Google Drive folder, offering an easy way to monitor improvements and share achievements with their families. This progress tracking not only makes the cognitive exercises more meaningful but also provides a sense of accomplishment for the people you support.

Last but not least, why not introduce a suite of apps designed specifically for older people and people with additional needs? Apps such as "Tell Me Wow Senior Games" offer a variety of games catering specifically to this demographic, further enhancing the accessibility and appeal of the Tiny Tablet's cognitive stimulation offerings.

In a nutshell, cognitive stimulation apps are more than just games; they're an engaging and fun tool to keep the minds sharp of the people you support. So, fire up the Tiny Tablet, let the brain games begin, and watch as your care setting turns into a lively hub of mental agility and friendly competition.

Chapter 17: Harnessing the Most Popular Activities for Optimal Engagement

Thrills and Skills: The Interactive Adventure of Games and Apps

Transform your care setting into an exciting arcade with a whole world of interactive games just a few taps away.

Using the Tiny Tablet, people can dive into a universe of fun, competing in everything from air hockey and chess to tennis and bowling. And to add that extra bit of excitement, setting up leaderboards can ignite a wave of friendly competition, creating a vibrant atmosphere of engagement and social interaction.

We're all familiar with the allure of games, their ability to pull us in and let us lose track of time. But with the Tiny Tablet, gaming becomes more than just a pastime. It becomes a way to improve reflexes, enhance strategic thinking, and boost the overall mood in the care setting. Each game becomes a new challenge to conquer, a new skill to master.

But let's not forget, games are also a fabulous way to stimulate social interaction. Whether it's a heated match of chess or a light-hearted round of air hockey, games encourage people to interact, collaborate, and maybe even indulge in a bit of playful banter. This heightened sense of community can significantly contribute to the mental and emotional wellbeing of the people you support.

Chapter 17: Harnessing the Most Popular Activities for Optimal Engagement

And now, let's bring on the leaderboards! Having a visual representation of everyone's scores can be a real game-changer.

Suddenly, there's a clear goal to strive for, a title to defend. And who doesn't love a bit of friendly competition? With leaderboards, you're not just keeping track of scores; you're fuelling motivation, encouraging participation, and generating a lively buzz around the Tiny Tablet.

Extend this idea further by hosting regular gaming tournaments. Imagine the excitement as people gather around to see who will be the reigning champion of the week in bowling or who has mastered the tricky moves in virtual tennis. These tournaments can become a highlight of the week, something people look forward to, instilling a sense of anticipation and excitement that goes beyond the games themselves.

And don't forget about the wide array of apps available for more personalised fun. Whether people enjoy strategy games, quizzes, puzzles, or even role-playing games, there's an app for that. These can be enjoyed individually or in groups, offering an immersive and engaging experience tailored to their interests.

In a nutshell, the interactive fun offered by games and apps on the Tiny Tablet is an adventure in itself. So, gear up, get gaming, and prepare to see your care setting brimming with energy, laughter, and a competitive spirit that brings everyone together!

Chapter 17: Harnessing the Most Popular Activities for Optimal Engagement

Mind-Bending Adventures: Diving Deep into Puzzle Games

Offer a world of mental stimulation to the people you support with the mesmerising allure of puzzle games. These mind-bending challenges are not only engaging but also encourage mental agility, quick reactions, and strategic thinking. From number games and word challenges to classic block games like Tetris or addictive match-three games like Candy Crush, there's a puzzle game for everyone. The Tiny Tablet becomes a portal to worlds that tickle the brain and keep people entertained for hours.

But puzzle games aren't just about individual enjoyment. They can become a group activity too. Staff can assist people who may need a little help navigating the games or join in the fun to create a lively and interactive experience. Maybe it's teaming up to solve a tricky crossword puzzle, or a collective effort to reach the next level in a number game – every interaction becomes an opportunity to bond, learn, and grow.

And to add an extra dash of excitement, why not track scores and progress? This gentle dose of friendly competition can stimulate the competitive spirit and encourage them to take on more challenges. After all, who doesn't enjoy the thrill of seeing their name at the top of the leaderboard? Celebrating these little victories can significantly boost confidence of the people you support and bring about a sense of accomplishment.

Chapter 17: Harnessing the Most Popular Activities for Optimal Engagement

Furthermore, consider having puzzle-solving sessions or themed puzzle days. Whether it's a Sunday Sudoku showdown or a mid-week mystery crossword event, these sessions can be both entertaining and cognitively enriching. Not to mention, they can offer a fresh break from the routine and keep those you care for looking forward to something new every week.

For people who may prefer a slower pace or something less competitive, serene puzzle games that allow them to work at their own rhythm are a great option. These can provide a calming and therapeutic effect while still engaging their minds in a fun and gentle way.

Let's not forget the tangible benefits of puzzle games. They promote problem-solving, improve memory, enhance focus, and can even slow cognitive decline. But at the end of the day, the joy of puzzle games lies in the journey, not just the destination. The eureka moments when a difficult puzzle is solved, the shared laughter when an answer seems elusive, the satisfaction of progress – these are the moments that truly encapsulate the joy of puzzle games.

So, get ready to turn your care setting into a puzzle-solving hub where every day brings new challenges to conquer, new victories to celebrate, and endless opportunities for mental growth and social interaction.

Chapter 17: Harnessing the Most Popular Activities for Optimal Engagement

Unlimited Imagination: Exploring Arts and Crafts Apps

Invite those you care for to immerse themselves in a world of creative possibilities with the diverse range of arts and crafts apps available on the Tiny Tablet. These apps are a beautiful amalgamation of art, technology, and imagination that provide an accessible and inclusive platform for everyone to express their creativity, regardless of their physical abilities.

From painting apps that turn the tablet into a canvas filled with vibrant colours, to virtual pottery apps that allow individuals to mould and decorate their own clay creations, there's an app for every artistic pursuit. With these, those you care for can explore different artistic mediums without worrying about the typical constraints of physical materials or clean-up afterwards.

Music lovers aren't left out either. With apps like Perfect Piano, they can learn to play musical instruments right on their tablets. These apps often come with tutorials and 'learn to play' sections, perfect for beginners or those looking to brush up on their skills.

Music can be a therapeutic and enriching experience, and these apps make it possible for everyone to enjoy and create music, regardless of their previous musical experience.

Chapter 17: Harnessing the Most Popular Activities for Optimal Engagement

Additionally, paint-by-number apps are an excellent choice for those who enjoy more structured art activities. These apps guide users to create stunning pictures by filling in numbered areas with specific colours. It's a calming, focused activity that combines the pleasure of colouring with the satisfaction of creating a beautiful picture that can be saved, shared, or even printed out.

And for those who enjoy the meticulous craft of cross-stitching but might find the physical process challenging due to limited hand mobility, there are virtual cross-stitch apps. These apps allow users to choose their patterns and colours, and then 'stitch' by tapping on the screen. This gives them the opportunity to engage in an activity they love, without the physical strain.

A group painting session or a communal pottery creation can be an enjoyable social activity that encourages interaction, collaboration, and the sharing of ideas and techniques. You could even host an 'art exhibition' where people can showcase their digital creations. These social events can create a sense of community, shared accomplishment, and pride.

The beauty of these arts and crafts apps is their accessibility and adaptability. They can cater to a wide variety of skill levels and interests, making them an inclusive activity for all people. So, encourage those you care for to express their inner Picasso, Beethoven, or Monet. Whether they are seasoned artists or trying their hand at art for the first time, these apps can provide hours of creative enjoyment and a beautiful outlet for self-expression. Let the artistic journey begin!

Chapter 17: Harnessing the Most Popular Activities for Optimal Engagement

In this exciting era of technological advancements, the possibilities to enhance quality of life and stimulate engagement for people in care settings are truly limitless. As we've explored in this chapter, the Internet and devices like the Tiny Tablet open up a whole new world of opportunities for both fun and learning.

From video calls that connect people with their loved ones and healthcare providers, to the immersive journeys offered by Google Earth, technology has the power to make individuals' worlds bigger, more connected, and more exciting.

Language learning and information exploration through platforms like YouTube and Wikipedia can stimulate cognitive abilities and encourage lifelong learning, while web browsing with Chrome and the use of sensory apps promote digital inclusion and well-being for all users.

The numerous games, brain-training exercises, puzzle-solving activities, and arts and crafts apps available transform the tablet into a versatile hub of engagement. Not only can these entertain and captivate the users, but they also promote social interaction, cognitive stimulation, problem-solving skills, and creative expression.

Chapter 17: Harnessing the Most Popular Activities for Optimal Engagement

Incorporating these digital tools and activities into your care setting can have a profound impact on the quality of life for the people you support. They offer both independent and communal experiences that can be tailored to individual interests and abilities.

In essence, it's about using technology as a means to an end, the end being the well-being and enrichment of people lives. It's all about embracing these opportunities for growth, learning, and joy that modern technology presents.

As we move forward, the world of digital engagement will only continue to evolve and expand, and we hope this guide has provided you with practical ways to harness the most popular activities for optimal engagement in your care setting. Now, it's time to dive in and start exploring these digital realms together!

Chapter 18: Enhancing Care with Music Therapy

The transformative power of music therapy has been recognised for centuries, and its potential to improve the lives of the older generations, particularly those living with dementia and Alzheimer's disease, is undeniable.

This guide will explore the various benefits of music therapy for people in care and how the Tiny Tablet touch screen activity table from www.inspired-inspirations.com can further amplify these benefits.

We will delve into the science behind music therapy, its impact on cognitive function, emotional well-being, and social connections, and how the innovative Tiny Tablet can make this therapeutic approach even more accessible and enjoyable for seniors in care settings.

Section 1: The Science of Music Therapy for Older People

1.1 Understanding the brain's response to music

Music has an extraordinary capacity to influence our emotions, memories, and even cognitive functions. This powerful effect can be attributed to the way our brains process music. When we listen to music, our brains engage multiple regions, including the auditory cortex, the limbic system (responsible for emotions), and the prefrontal cortex (involved in planning and decision-making).

Chapter 18: Enhancing Care with Music Therapy

Additionally, music stimulates the release of neurotransmitters such as dopamine, which plays a crucial role in reward and pleasure sensations, and oxytocin, often referred to as the "love hormone" for its role in social bonding. This complex interplay between brain regions and neurotransmitters allows music to impact our mental and emotional well-being profoundly.

1.2 Music therapy's effects on cognitive function in dementia and Alzheimer's patients

For people living with dementia and Alzheimer's disease, music therapy offers a promising approach to enhancing cognitive function. Research has shown that music can stimulate the brain in ways that other interventions may not, primarily because it engages multiple neural networks, even those that may be unaffected by neurodegenerative diseases.

A study conducted by the National Institute for Stroke and Applied Neurosciences in New Zealand demonstrated that music therapy could improve memory recall and recognition in patients with dementia. This can be attributed to the involvement of the temporal lobe, which plays a significant role in memory and emotional processing, in the brain's response to music.

Chapter 18: Enhancing Care with Music Therapy

Moreover, music therapy can also enhance other cognitive functions such as attention, executive function, and visuospatial skills. This comprehensive cognitive improvement can contribute to a better quality of life and reduced caregiver burden for people living with dementia and Alzheimer's.

1.3 Music therapy as an emotional support for people living with neurodegenerative disorders

People living with dementia and Alzheimer's often experience emotional challenges such as anxiety, depression, and agitation. Music therapy can provide emotional support for these people by offering a non-verbal means of communication and self-expression. Through music, they can convey their feelings, even when verbal communication becomes challenging.

By providing a soothing and familiar environment, music therapy can help reduce agitation, stress, and anxiety. Familiar songs or melodies can evoke positive emotions and memories, providing comfort and a sense of identity for people living with neurodegenerative disorders.

Chapter 18: Enhancing Care with Music Therapy

Furthermore, music therapy can also enhance self-esteem and overall well-being by allowing people to participate in a meaningful activity. Engaging in music therapy can offer a sense of accomplishment and purpose, essential for maintaining emotional health and quality of life.

The science behind music therapy for older people underscores its potential to improve cognitive function and provide emotional support for individuals living with dementia and Alzheimer's.

By understanding the brain's response to music and its role in enhancing cognition and emotional well-being, caregivers and care facilities can harness the power of music therapy to offer a more comprehensive and compassionate approach to care.

Chapter 18: Enhancing Care with Music Therapy

Section 2: Music Therapy and Emotional Well-being

2.1 Addressing depression and anxiety in older people living with dementia and Alzheimer's through music therapy.

Depression and anxiety are common emotional challenges faced by people with dementia and Alzheimer's. Music therapy can be an effective tool in addressing these issues by providing a safe, non-pharmacological, and non-invasive intervention.

A study conducted by the University of Kansas found that music therapy significantly reduced symptoms of depression and anxiety in people living with dementia. The therapeutic benefits of music can be attributed to its ability to stimulate the release of neurotransmitters such as serotonin and dopamine, which play a crucial role in regulating mood and emotions.

Furthermore, music therapy provides a comforting and familiar environment that can help people living with dementia and Alzheimer's feel more at ease. Familiar songs and melodies can evoke positive emotions and memories, offering a sense of connection to their past and identity.

This sense of familiarity and comfort can alleviate anxiety and foster a sense of emotional stability.

Chapter 18: Enhancing Care with Music Therapy

2.2 The power of music in evoking memories and emotions

One of the most remarkable aspects of music therapy is its ability to evoke memories and emotions, even in people with advanced stages of dementia and Alzheimer's. Music has a unique capacity to tap into the emotional memory system, which is often less affected by neurodegenerative diseases than other memory systems.

When people listen to familiar music from their past, it can stimulate the emotional memory system, evoking feelings of nostalgia, happiness, and even sadness. These emotional responses can create a powerful sense of connection and belonging, which is essential for maintaining emotional well-being and combating feelings of isolation and loneliness.

Moreover, music can serve as a bridge between people living with dementia and Alzheimer's and their caregivers or loved ones.

Sharing memories and emotions evoked by music can facilitate communication and bonding, providing an invaluable source of emotional support and connection.

Chapter 18: Enhancing Care with Music Therapy

2.3 The role of music therapy in enhancing mood and overall well-being

Music therapy plays a vital role in enhancing mood and overall well-being for people living with dementia and Alzheimer's. By offering an engaging, enjoyable, and meaningful activity, music therapy can contribute to a sense of purpose and accomplishment, which is crucial for maintaining self-esteem and well-being.

Additionally, the positive emotions and memories evoked by music can help improve mood and foster a sense of happiness and contentment. A study conducted by the University of Utah found that music therapy significantly improved the mood and well-being of people living with dementia, as it stimulates parts of the brain that remain unaffected by the disease.

Music therapy is a powerful tool for enhancing emotional well-being in seniors with dementia and Alzheimer's. By addressing depression and anxiety, evoking memories and emotions, and improving mood and overall well-being, music therapy offers a holistic and compassionate approach to care that can significantly improve the quality of life for those living with neurodegenerative disorders.

Chapter 18: Enhancing Care with Music Therapy

Section 3: The Tiny Tablet Touch Screen Activity Table: A Game-Changer in Music Therapy For Older People

3.1 The innovative features of the Tiny Tablet touch screen activity table

The Tiny Tablet touch screen activity table from www.inspired-inspirations.com is an innovative device designed to enhance the music therapy experience for people. Combining cutting-edge technology with user-friendly features, the Tiny Tablet offers a versatile and engaging platform for seniors to explore music therapy in a fun and interactive way.

Equipped with apps such as YouTube and Spotify, the Tiny Tablet allows people to enjoy a wide range of music from different genres and eras. The touch screen technology enables people to easily control the music, making the experience more immersive and enjoyable. Furthermore, the adjustable height and angle of the table ensure that seniors with limited mobility can access the device comfortably and safely.

3.2 Empowering seniors through easy access to music therapy

One of the most significant advantages of the Tiny Tablet touch screen activity table is its ability to empower people by providing easy access to music therapy. The touch screen interface allows people to search for and play their favourite songs without the need for assistance, which can be particularly empowering for those with limited mobility or cognitive abilities.

Chapter 18: Enhancing Care with Music Therapy

By enabling people you support to control their own music choices, the Tiny Tablet fosters a sense of independence and autonomy that can contribute to improved self-esteem and well-being. Additionally, the device offers people the opportunity to explore new music and rediscover old favourites, further enhancing their music therapy experience.

3.3 Promoting a sense of purpose and independence for older people with limited mobility and cognitive abilities

For people with limited mobility and cognitive abilities, the Tiny Tablet touch screen activity table offers an opportunity to engage in music therapy in a way that promotes a sense of purpose and independence. By allowing people to control their own music choices, the Tiny Tablet provides them with a meaningful activity that can help combat feelings of isolation, boredom, and frustration.

Moreover, the Tiny Tablet's touch screen technology is designed to be accessible and easy to use, even for people with cognitive impairments or limited motor skills. This ensures that they can participate in music therapy without the need for constant assistance, thereby promoting a sense of independence and control over their own experiences.

By embracing the Tiny Tablet and music therapy, caregivers can provide a comprehensive and compassionate approach to care that supports cognitive function, emotional well-being, and social connections.

Chapter 18: Enhancing Care with Music Therapy

Section 4: Music Therapy as a Catalyst for Social Connections

4.1 Fostering social interaction and community-building through shared musical experiences

Music therapy can serve as an effective catalyst for social connections among people, particularly those in care settings. Shared musical experiences provide common ground for people to engage in conversations and activities, fostering social interaction and community-building. By participating in group music therapy sessions or listening to music together, people can develop bonds and forge new friendships based on their mutual appreciation for music.

In addition to group activities, the Tiny Tablet touch screen activity table can also facilitate social connections by allowing people to share their favourite songs, exchange stories about concerts or musical memories, and explore new music together. These shared experiences can help create a sense of camaraderie and unity among those in care, contributing to a more positive and supportive care environment.

4.2 Breaking down barriers and combating isolation in care settings

Social isolation and loneliness are common challenges faced by those in care settings, particularly those with dementia and Alzheimer's who may struggle with communication and memory loss. Music therapy can play a crucial role in breaking down barriers and combating isolation by providing a non-verbal means of communication and shared interest.

Chapter 18: Enhancing Care with Music Therapy

The emotional power of music allows people to connect with others on a deeper level, transcending the limitations imposed by cognitive decline or communication difficulties.

Through music, people can express themselves, share memories, and connect with their peers in a meaningful way, mitigating feelings of isolation and loneliness.

The Tiny Tablet touch screen activity table can further enhance social connections by providing an accessible platform for people to engage with music and interact with one another. The device's user-friendly interface enables people with varying levels of cognitive and physical abilities to participate in music therapy, ensuring that no one is left out of the social benefits it offers.

4.3 Providing a sense of purpose and belonging through music-related discussions and activities

Music therapy can provide people with a sense of purpose and belonging by offering opportunities for music-related discussions and activities. Engaging in conversations about favourite songs, artists, or concerts can help people feel valued and connected to their community, fostering a sense of belonging and well-being.

Chapter 18: Enhancing Care with Music Therapy

In addition to discussions, music therapy can also involve collaborative activities such as singing, playing instruments, or even composing songs. These activities provide people with a sense of accomplishment and purpose, contributing to their overall emotional and mental well-being.

By incorporating the Tiny Tablet touch screen activity table into music therapy sessions, caregivers can create a dynamic and engaging environment for people to explore their musical interests and connect with others.

This can lead to a greater sense of purpose and belonging, essential components of a positive and supportive care experience.

Music therapy serves as a powerful catalyst for social connections among people, particularly in care settings. By fostering social interaction, breaking down barriers, and providing a sense of purpose and belonging, music therapy contributes to a more positive and inclusive care environment that supports the emotional and mental well-being of all people being supported.

The Tiny Tablet touch screen activity table further enhances these benefits, ensuring that people have the tools and resources they need to fully engage in the transformative power of music therapy.

Chapter 18: Enhancing Care with Music Therapy

Section 5: Music Therapy and the Future of Social Care

5.1 Integrating music therapy into holistic care plans for people being supported

As the benefits of music therapy become increasingly recognised, integrating it into holistic care plans for people is essential. A comprehensive care plan that considers the physical, cognitive, emotional, and social needs of individuals can significantly improve their overall well-being and quality of life.

Incorporating music therapy into these plans can address several of these needs simultaneously, making it a valuable component of comprehensive senior care.

Caregivers, healthcare professionals, and family members should work together to identify the most effective ways to incorporate music therapy into individuals' daily routines.

This can include group music therapy sessions, individualised music playlists, or access to devices like the Tiny Tablet touch screen activity table to facilitate self-directed music therapy experiences.

Chapter 18: Enhancing Care with Music Therapy

5.2 The potential of emerging technologies in enhancing music therapy experiences

As technology continues to advance, there is significant potential for emerging technologies to enhance music therapy experiences for people in supported care. Devices like the Tiny Tablet touch screen activity table are just the beginning; future innovations could include virtual reality experiences that immerse people in musical environments or artificial intelligence systems that can create personalised music therapy sessions based on a persons preferences and needs.

By embracing these emerging technologies, caregivers and care settings can provide even more engaging and effective music therapy experiences. This not only improves the quality of care but also offers people new and exciting ways to explore their musical interests and connect with others.

5.3 The importance of continued research and innovation in music therapy for older people

As our understanding of the benefits of music therapy for people continues to grow, it is crucial to support ongoing research and innovation in this field. This includes studies examining the long-term effects of music therapy on cognitive function and emotional well-being, as well as research exploring the potential benefits of music therapy for people with other conditions, such as Parkinson's disease or stroke.

Chapter 18: Enhancing Care with Music Therapy

Supporting this research can lead to new discoveries and breakthroughs that will further enhance the effectiveness of music therapy for people in care.

Additionally, investing in innovation can help develop new tools, technologies, and approaches to music therapy, ensuring that people continue to have access to the most effective and engaging therapeutic experiences possible.

Chapter 19: Implementing Talking Therapy in Care via Apps

Talking therapy can have transformative impacts on the mental health of older people. Despite societal stereotypes suggesting mental health is secondary to physical health in older adults, research and real-world experiences reveal that conversing about mental health can significantly improve the quality of life for people in aged care.

Unfortunately, many older adults fail to seek help due to misconceptions about mental health being a natural part of ageing.

However, innovative technology solutions such as the Tiny Tablet touch screen activity tables and app-based technology are striving to change this narrative.

The Importance of Talking Therapy in Care

As Heather Stonebank, Lead Psychological Wellbeing Practitioner (PWP) for the NHS Improving Access to Psychological Therapies (IAPT) program highlights, talking therapy has the potential to bring about profound change.

The IAPT program aims to help people overcome depression and anxiety, with a focus on older adults in recent years. While there has been a rise in older adults accessing these treatments, they are still underrepresented. The reasons vary from misconceptions about mental health issues in older people to a lack of knowledge about the help available.

Chapter 19: Implementing Talking Therapy in Care via Apps

Talking therapy is vital as we age, as it helps manage both mental and physical health. It is a collaborative process where the patient, being an expert in themselves, works with the therapist to choose the best treatment that can be adapted to their individual needs.

Older people typically respond well to talking therapy, with high commitment levels and willingness to try new techniques.

A Novel Approach

In this digital age, the potential to transform mental health care for older adults has never been more promising. Tiny Tablet touch screen activity tables and app-based technology introduce a modern and engaging approach to stimulate conversations and interactions among those in care.

The Tiny Tablet touch screen activity tables are specially designed for user-friendly interaction, providing an easy-to-use interface for older people who may not be familiar with digital technology. This technology incorporates features such as large, clear buttons and adjustable text sizes, making it accessible to users with varying levels of visual acuity and digital proficiency.

The touch screen interface offers a tactile experience, encouraging active engagement and interaction with the content.

Chapter 19: Implementing Talking Therapy in Care via Apps

App-based technology further enhances this experience by providing diverse and dynamic content. The integration of popular apps like Google Earth, YouTube, Wikipedia, Spotify, and Google Chrome significantly enhances the conversation points, stimulating the minds of the people you support and encouraging them to engage in discussions.

Google Earth: A Gateway to Reminiscence and Connection in Care

Google Earth's digital platform offers a unique, interactive tool for facilitating reminiscence therapy among those in care. By virtually transporting users to any corner of the globe, it stimulates a sense of adventure and curiosity, evokes potent memories, and encourages vibrant discussions that can significantly enhance mental wellbeing.

Our emotional connections to places play a significant role in shaping our identities and memories. Revisiting these places, even virtually, can elicit strong emotional responses, triggering a wave of nostalgia and remembrance. For people in care, this can mean revisiting their childhood homes, the streets they used to roam, the parks where they played, or the cities where they raised their families.

These experiences can bring immense joy and comfort, alleviating feelings of isolation or loneliness that some people may experience. Moreover, this journey down memory lane provides an opportunity to relive happy times, fostering a positive mental state and enhancing overall wellbeing.

Chapter 19: Implementing Talking Therapy in Care via Apps

Google Earth's virtual tours also provide a platform for people to share their life stories and experiences. As they navigate the streets of their past, they can share tales of their youth, adventures, hardships, and triumphs.

These stories not only stimulate meaningful conversations but also create a sense of community and understanding among individuals. Hearing about others' experiences and sharing their own can help people feel valued, heard, and connected, promoting emotional wellbeing.

Beyond reminiscing about the past, Google Earth also allows people to explore new places they've always wished to visit. Whether it's the Eiffel Tower in Paris, the Great Wall of China, or the Grand Canyon in Arizona, people can embark on virtual adventures from the comfort of their care setting.

This sense of exploration and discovery can have profound emotional benefits. It can instil a sense of excitement and wonder, combat feelings of stagnation, and even inspire individuals to dream and set new goals.

It also provides a shared experience that can serve as a conversation starter, fostering social connections and stimulating mental engagement.

Chapter 19: Implementing Talking Therapy in Care via Apps

Through Google Earth, individuals can virtually visit different cultures and societies around the world, fostering empathy and understanding. This global perspective encourages open-mindedness and respect for diversity, which are beneficial for creating a harmonious community environment within the care setting.

Moreover, understanding and appreciating different cultures can promote a sense of connectedness and solidarity, contributing to emotional wellbeing.

Incorporating Google Earth into the Tiny Tablet touch screen activity tables is more than just providing entertainment; it's about creating opportunities for emotional engagement, social connection, intellectual stimulation, and personal growth.

This app-based technology can play a critical role in promoting mental health among people in care, demonstrating the power of technology in enhancing the quality of life.

Chapter 19: Implementing Talking Therapy in Care via Apps

YouTube: Fostering Connection, Engagement, and Joy in Care

YouTube, with its virtually limitless library of audio-visual content, offers a uniquely versatile platform for facilitating interaction and emotional engagement among people in care settings. From music videos and documentaries to DIY tutorials and comedy sketches, YouTube caters to diverse interests and preferences, fostering social bonds, stimulating intellectual curiosity, and promoting emotional wellbeing.

One of the main benefits of YouTube lies in its ability to bring people together over shared interests. The platform offers content on virtually any topic imaginable, enabling people with similar interests to come together and enjoy shared experiences. Whether it's watching a classic movie, enjoying a concert of a beloved band, or learning about gardening techniques, these shared activities can lead to deeper connections and stronger bonds.

The simple act of watching a video together can trigger discussions, debates, and shared laughter, enhancing social interaction and contributing to a sense of community.

As people connect over shared interests, they feel more understood and less alone, boosting their overall emotional wellbeing.

Chapter 19: Implementing Talking Therapy in Care via Apps

YouTube hosts a rich collection of vintage music, movies, and TV shows, offering a powerful tool for reminiscence therapy.

People can relive cherished memories by watching content from their younger years, evoking emotions of nostalgia and joy. A song from a particular era, for example, might bring back memories of special events, past relationships, or significant life milestones.

Reminiscing over these memories can evoke a range of emotions and stimulate personal storytelling, where people share their past experiences and life stories. This not only promotes emotional expression but also strengthens intergenerational understanding and empathy among people, fostering a more supportive and inclusive community.

YouTube is also a valuable resource for lifelong learning. The platform offers educational content on a wide range of subjects, from history and science to arts and crafts. By watching documentaries or tutorials, people can continue to learn and grow, keeping their minds active and engaged.

The act of learning stimulates intellectual curiosity and promotes mental flexibility, both of which are beneficial for cognitive health. Moreover, learning new skills or gaining new knowledge can enhance self-esteem and provide a sense of accomplishment, contributing to overall emotional wellbeing.

Chapter 19: Implementing Talking Therapy in Care via Apps

The power of laughter and entertainment in promoting mental health cannot be understated, and YouTube is a treasure trove of humorous and entertaining content. Watching comedy sketches or funny animal videos, for example, can provide much-needed laughter and joy, acting as a natural stress reliever.

Laughter promotes the release of endorphins, the body's natural feel-good chemicals, leading to feelings of happiness and relaxation. It also brings people together, fostering a sense of camaraderie and shared joy among people in care.

Incorporating YouTube into the digital resources of care settings via Tiny Tablet touch screen activity tables has the potential to significantly enhance the quality of life for those in care.

Its diverse content caters to various interests and emotional needs, promoting social connection, intellectual engagement, emotional expression, and above all, joy. As such, YouTube serves as an invaluable tool in promoting mental health and emotional wellbeing in care.

Chapter 19: Implementing Talking Therapy in Care via Apps

Wikipedia: Stimulating Lifelong Learning and Community in Aged Care

Wikipedia, the online encyclopaedia, is a comprehensive resource that can stimulate intellectual curiosity and facilitate lifelong learning among people in care. With articles on virtually every conceivable topic, from history and science to arts and culture, Wikipedia provides a platform for enriching discussions, fostering a sense of community, and enhancing emotional wellbeing among those in care settings.

Lifelong learning is a critical aspect of mental health and wellbeing in care. The process of learning keeps the mind active and engaged, helping to maintain cognitive abilities and even slow the progression of cognitive decline.

Wikipedia, with its vast repository of knowledge, offers an excellent tool for fostering this continual learning.

People can delve into articles about historical events, explore scientific concepts, or learn about different cultures and societies. This intellectual stimulation not only keeps the mind active but also fosters a sense of curiosity and wonder, combating feelings of boredom or stagnation that can sometimes occur in care settings.

Chapter 19: Implementing Talking Therapy in Care via Apps

Exploring Wikipedia articles can also serve as a social activity, fostering connections among people.

As they delve into topics of shared interest, they can engage in lively discussions, debate ideas, and share their insights. These interactions can create a sense of community, mitigating feelings of isolation and loneliness.

For example, a group of people interested in gardening might explore Wikipedia articles about different plant species, gardening techniques, or the history of gardening. This shared learning experience can lead to enriching conversations and even inspire group activities, such as starting a community garden in the facility.

Wikipedia can also contribute to enhancing self-esteem and feelings of empowerment. The ability to learn new information, understand complex topics, and engage in intellectual conversations can provide a sense of accomplishment and purpose.

In care settings, it's common for people to feel a loss of control or independence. However, the act of self-directed learning through Wikipedia can help restore a sense of agency and autonomy. This, in turn, can contribute to improved mood, increased motivation, and a more positive outlook.

Chapter 19: Implementing Talking Therapy in Care via Apps

Finally, the wealth of information available on Wikipedia can foster empathy and cultural understanding. By exploring articles about different cultures, societies, and historical events, individuals can gain a broader perspective on the world. This can promote open-mindedness, understanding, and respect for diversity, which are essential for creating a harmonious and inclusive community within the aged care facility.

The integration of Wikipedia into the Tiny Tablet touch screen activity tables within care settings can offer significant benefits. From stimulating lifelong learning and fostering community connections to enhancing self-esteem and promoting cultural understanding,

Wikipedia is an invaluable tool for promoting mental health and emotional wellbeing. As such, it stands as an example of how technology can be harnessed to enhance the quality of life in care.

Chapter 19: Implementing Talking Therapy in Care via Apps

Spotify: Harnessing the Power of Music in Care

Spotify, with its extensive library of music spanning various genres and eras, offers a unique tool for fostering emotional engagement and social interaction among people in care settings. Music has the power to touch our souls, evoke emotions, and stimulate memories. Through shared listening experiences, impromptu dance parties, or quiet moments of reflection, Spotify can contribute to creating a joyful and connected community, thereby promoting emotional wellbeing.

Music has a profound connection with memory. A familiar melody or a certain song can transport us back in time, triggering vivid memories of people, places, and events from our past. For those in care, Spotify's vast music library can serve as a conduit for reminiscence therapy.

People can listen to the songs of their youth, reliving memories and sharing their stories with others.

This can lead to deep, heartfelt conversations, strengthening social bonds and fostering a sense of belonging. Moreover, the act of reminiscing can have therapeutic benefits, providing comfort, enhancing mood, and improving overall emotional wellbeing.

Chapter 19: Implementing Talking Therapy in Care via Apps

Group music listening sessions using Spotify can create a joyful and lively atmosphere within the care setting. Whether it's a shared appreciation for classical symphonies, a communal sing-along to old-time favourites, or even a dance party to a rocking playlist, these shared experiences can bring people together, encouraging them to open up and connect with each other.

Music can serve as a universal language, transcending barriers and fostering shared enjoyment. These joyful experiences can significantly enhance a persons' mood, alleviate feelings of loneliness, and promote a sense of community.

Spotify also allows people to express their individuality and preferences. Each person can curate their personal playlists, choosing songs that hold special meaning for them or simply align with their musical tastes.

This act of personal expression can provide a sense of autonomy and control, which are crucial for emotional wellbeing in care settings.

Moreover, sharing their personal playlists with others allows people to reveal aspects of their identity and life story, fostering understanding and mutual respect among those in care.

Chapter 19: Implementing Talking Therapy in Care via Apps

Music can also be a powerful tool for emotional wellbeing. Listening to music can have a calming effect, reducing stress and anxiety, and promoting relaxation. For people dealing with emotional challenges, music can serve as a form of solace, offering comfort and emotional release.

On the other hand, upbeat and lively music can lift spirits, energise the atmosphere, and inspire positivity. Whether it's through soothing melodies or invigorating rhythms, music can significantly influence mood and emotional state.

Incorporating Spotify into the Tiny Tablet touch screen activity tables provides a valuable resource for emotional engagement, social connection, personal expression, and joy within care settings. By harnessing the power of music, Spotify serves as a potent tool for enhancing emotional wellbeing and quality of life among those in care.

This is a testament to the transformative potential of app-based technology in care, as it brings joy, connection, and emotional richness into the lives of individuals.

Chapter 19: Implementing Talking Therapy in Care via Apps

Google Chrome: Fostering Exploration and Connection in Care

Google Chrome, as a versatile and user-friendly web browser, serves as a gateway to the vast world of online resources. It provides countless opportunities for exploration, learning, and engagement for people in care settings. Whether it's reading news articles, exploring hobbies, joining online communities, or just surfing the web, Google Chrome can stimulate thought-provoking conversations, promote social interaction, and enhance mental wellbeing.

The internet, accessible via Google Chrome, is a treasure trove of information and resources on virtually any topic imaginable.

People can read up on current events, research topics of interest, explore hobbies, or learn new skills. This continuous learning and exploration help keep the mind active and engaged, contributing to cognitive health.

For instance, people you support who are interested in art could explore online galleries or read up on different art movements and techniques. Meanwhile, another person might enjoy keeping up with current events and sharing their insights with others. These activities not only stimulate intellectual engagement but also foster a sense of curiosity and personal growth.

Chapter 19: Implementing Talking Therapy in Care via Apps

Google Chrome can also facilitate social connections among those in care. As they explore their interests online, people can share their findings with each other, leading to enriching discussions and shared experiences.

For example, someone might discover an interesting article or video and share it with others. This can spark lively debates, shared laughter, or deep reflections, helping to strengthen social bonds and build a sense of community.

Through Google Chrome, people can also stay connected with the wider world. They can read news from their hometowns, follow global events, or even join online communities related to their interests.

Being part of these online communities can provide a sense of belonging and help combat feelings of isolation. It can also foster a sense of understanding and empathy as people engage with diverse perspectives and experiences from around the world.

The ability to navigate the internet through Google Chrome can also foster a sense of empowerment and autonomy among people. In a care setting, where people may often feel a loss of independence, being able to explore the online world at their own pace and according to their interests can restore a sense of control and agency. This can significantly enhance their self-esteem and overall emotional wellbeing.

Chapter 19: Implementing Talking Therapy in Care via Apps

Google Chrome, as an integral part of the Tiny Tablet touch screen activity tables, offers immense potential for promoting mental wellbeing in care settings.

By fostering exploration, lifelong learning, social connections, and a sense of empowerment, Google Chrome serves as an invaluable tool for enhancing the quality of life for those in care.

As such, it exemplifies the transformative potential of app-based technology in care, offering people the opportunity to engage with the world in meaningful and enriching ways.

Chapter 19: Implementing Talking Therapy in Care via Apps

Embracing Technology for Emotional Wellbeing in Care

Mental health is as important as physical health in care, and talking therapy serves as a vital instrument in its management. In the digital age, the potential to leverage technology, such as Tiny Tablet touch screen activity tables and app-based tools, allows you to enhance the reach and impact of these therapeutic methods.

Each of the apps we've discussed—Google Earth, YouTube, Wikipedia, Spotify, and Google Chrome—offers unique ways to stimulate conversation, foster connections, and promote emotional wellbeing among people in care settings.

These apps, when used collaboratively on the Tiny Tablet touch screen activity tables, create a dynamic and interactive environment. They foster a sense of community among the people you support, providing them with shared experiences that stimulate conversation and deepen connections. They also provide opportunities for people to express their individuality, explore their interests, and engage with the world in a way that is meaningful to them.

This integration of technology into talking therapy in care not only enhances the effectiveness of therapeutic interventions but also improves the quality of life for people. It empowers them to take an active role in managing their mental health, encouraging autonomy, continuous learning, and social engagement.

Chapter 20: Uncovering the Impact of Tiny Tablet Activity Tables on Well-being

In the era of rapid technological advancement, the intersection of technology and care has become an exciting realm to explore.

The Tiny Tablet Touch Screen Activity Table is one such innovative tool designed to revolutionise the experience of people you support, bringing about significant improvements to their overall well-being.

Promoting Social Interaction

One of the most remarkable effects of the Tiny Tablet activity tables on well-being is their capacity to encourage social interaction.

With an array of games and group activities, these tables transform solitary experiences into shared ones, encouraging users to play together, compete, and enjoy shared experiences.

In many care settings, social isolation can be a significant problem. The introduction of these interactive tables can foster a sense of community and camaraderie among people, as they gather around to engage in group activities or simply to watch and cheer on their peers.

As a result, these tablets can act as a catalyst to strengthen social bonds and diminish feelings of loneliness, which is crucial for mental well-being.

Chapter 20: Uncovering the Impact of Tiny Tablet Activity Tables on Well-being

Cognitive Stimulation

The Tiny Tablet isn't just a hub of entertainment; it's a gymnasium for the mind. With a variety of brain-training apps and games designed specifically to boost cognitive function, these activity tables can contribute significantly to maintaining and even enhancing cognitive health.

Puzzle games, trivia quizzes, memory exercises, and problem-solving tasks all offer opportunities to exercise different cognitive functions such as memory, attention, problem-solving, and speed of processing. They provide a stimulating and enjoyable way for people to keep their minds active and sharp, which can be particularly beneficial for those with dementia or cognitive impairments.

Encouraging Physical Activity

While touch screen activity tables may seem unlikely tools for promoting physical activity, they can play a surprisingly effective role in encouraging people to engage in gentle physical exercise. Some games require hand-eye coordination, and the action of touching or swiping the screen can aid in maintaining fine motor skills.

In addition, some applications encourage more extensive physical engagement. For instance, certain virtual reality (VR) games might require users to 'swim' with their arms or 'walk' with their hands, promoting low-impact physical exercise, all while providing an immersive and entertaining experience.

Chapter 20: Uncovering the Impact of Tiny Tablet Activity Tables on Well-being

Emotional Well-being and Relaxation

The Tiny Tablet isn't just for games and learning; it also offers an array of apps and features designed to promote relaxation and emotional well-being. Apps with soothing nature sounds, calming visuals, and guided meditations can help to reduce anxiety and promote relaxation. Art and music apps provide a creative outlet for self-expression and can be incredibly therapeutic. They can offer immense satisfaction, from the joy of creating a digital painting to the serenity of playing a virtual piano. Such activities can boost mood, alleviate stress, and provide a sense of accomplishment, thereby enhancing emotional well-being.

Facilitating Communication

In the digital age, staying connected is easier than ever. The Tiny Tablet Activity Tables can be instrumental in helping people in care stay connected with their families and friends. Whether it's through video calls, sharing photos, or even playing online multiplayer games with their loved ones, these touch screen tables can play a crucial role in facilitating communication and maintaining strong relationships, which contributes positively to the persons' emotional health.

Tiny Tablet Touch Screen Activity Tables have shown to have a multifaceted impact on well-being, addressing aspects of social, cognitive, physical, and emotional health. By presenting a multitude of engagement opportunities in an accessible, user-friendly format, they significantly enrich the care setting experience.

Chapter 21: "My Story So Far" Fact-Finding Questionnaire

As we walk along the path of life, the journey we traverse is uniquely our own, marked by personal experiences, learnings, growth, and evolution. In the context of care, comprehending each persons' journey becomes crucial, not just to deliver personalised care but also to appreciate the progress they make, the milestones they achieve, and the challenges they overcome. The "My Story So Far" fact-finding initiative serves as a tool to chronicle these individual journeys and to illuminate the way forward.

The "My Story So Far" initiative can have a multifaceted impact. For one, it assists in creating a personalised well-being plan tailored to each persons' needs, strengths, and preferences. It facilitates an understanding of how far the person has come in their journey, offering valuable insights that guide the next steps for supported care.

Moreover, this narrative approach can be incredibly empowering for people themselves.

Sharing their stories, reminiscing about their past, and recognising their growth can promote a sense of identity, dignity, and self-esteem. It's not just about documenting where they are but also about celebrating who they are and what they've achieved.

Chapter 21: "My Story So Far" Fact-Finding Questionnaire

The questionnaire is designed to capture a comprehensive picture of each persons experiences and progress. It encourages respondents to reflect on various aspects of their lives, ranging from personal history and significant life events to their experiences and their aspirations for the future.

The questions are structured to elicit both factual information and personal reflections. They delve into areas such as cognitive function, social interactions, emotional well-being, and personal interests.

Through the answers, care providers can gain a rich understanding of the person behind the individual - their past, their present, and their potential. By tracking these responses over time, they can also document the individuals progress and adapt their care strategies accordingly.

MY STORY SO FAR

PICTURE

MY NAME IS

....

YOU CAN CALL ME

....

D.O.B. ....

BIRTH PLACE ....

I GREW UP IN .... ON .... ROAD

I WENT TO .... SCHOOL

MY MOTHERS NAME ....

MY FATHERS NAME ....

MY BROTHERS/SISTERS

....
....
....
....

MY STORY SO FAR

THE MOST FUN PARTS OF GROWING UP FOR ME WERE

....
....
....
....

MY FAVOURITE PLACE TO GO AS A CHILD WAS

....
....
....
....

MY FAVOURITE HOBBY AS A CHILD WAS

....
....
....
....

AS A CHILD I WAS PARTICULARLY GOOD AT

....
....
....
....

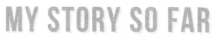

MY STORY SO FAR

MY FIRST JOB WAS

....

....

....

....

MY FAVOURITE JOB WAS

....

....

....

....

MY LAST JOB WAS

....

....

....

....

IF I WAS TO GO BACK TO WORK NOW I WOULD BE A

....

....

....

....

MY STORY SO FAR

I MET MY HUSBAND/WIFE AT

....
....
....
....

WE GOT MARRIED AT .... AND THE BEST WAY TO
DESCRIBE THE DAY WAS ....
....
....
....
....
....

WE HAVE .... CHILDREN AND .... GRANDCHILDREN. THEY ARE NAMED

....
....
....
....
....
....

MY STORY SO FAR

MY FAVOURITE SPORTS ARE

....
....
....
....

THE SPORTS TEAMS I FOLLOW ARE

....
....
....
....
....

MY FAVOURITE SPORTING MATCHES ARE

....
....
....
....

MY FAVOURITE SPORTING HERO IS

....
....
....
....

MY STORY SO FAR

MY FAVOURITE ANIMALS ARE

....
....
....
....

THE ANIMALS I WISH I'D SEEN IN REAL LIFE ARE

....
....
....
....

THE PETS I HAVE HAD ARE

....
....
....
....
....
....
....
....
....

MY STORY SO FAR

MY CLOSE FAMILY LIVE

....

....

....

....

....

....

MY FAVOURITE PLACE TO GO ON HOLIDAY IN THE UK IS

....

....

....

....

MY FAVOURITE PLACE TO GO ON HOLIDAY OUT OF THE UK IS

....

....

....

....

THE ONE PLACE I WISH I HAD VISITED IS

....

....

....

....

MY STORY SO FAR

MY TOP 3 PASSIONS OR HOBBIES ARE

....
....
....
....
....
....
....

MY FAVOURITE FOODS AND DRINKS ARE

....
....
....
....

MY FAVOURITE MUSIC/ARTISTS ARE

....
....
....
....

MY FAVOURITE COMEDIANS ARE

....
....
....
....
....

MY STORY SO FAR

MY FAVOURITE FILMS ARE

....

....

....

....

MY FAVOURITE TV PROGRAMMES ARE

....

....

....

....

MY FAVOURITE BOOKS ARE

....

....

....

....

MY FAVOURITE WAYS TO RELAX ARE

....

....

....

....

MY STORY SO FAR

IF I COULD LEARN A NEW SKILL IT WOULD BE

....
....
....
....

IF I COULD LEARN A NEW LANGUAGE IT WOULD BE

....
....
....
....

IF I COULD LEARN ABOUT ANY TOPIC IT WOULD BE

....
....
....
....

IF I COULD DEVELOP A NEW HOBBY IT WOULD BE

....
....
....
....

Chapter 21: "My Story So Far" Fact-Finding Questionnaire

In essence, the "My Story So Far" fact-finding initiative is more than a simple tool for documentation. It's a window into the lives of the people you support, offering a glimpse of their journey, their struggles, their victories, and their unique identities.

By recognising and honouring each person's story, we can foster a sense of belonging, respect, and individuality within the care environment. We can create a space where every voice is heard, every story matters, and every journey is celebrated.

It is indeed a powerful tool, one that can serve to enhance the overall quality of care provided and enrich the lives of those residing within care homes.

As we move forward, the "My Story So Far" initiative will continue to be instrumental in fostering a deeper understanding of each individual and their unique journey, paving the way for more personalised, compassionate, and effective care.

Chapter 22: Integrating Technology in Care Collaboration

Community involvement in care settings is a cornerstone for fostering a sense of belonging, stimulating social interactions, and promoting overall well-being among people you support.

The advent of technology has opened new avenues for integrating the local community into the care environment. In this chapter, we will explore how a Tiny Tablet can act as a tool for community connection, facilitating a wide range of interactions from intergenerational bonds to spiritual engagements.

Engaging the Young Generation

A Tiny Tablet can serve as a bridge between generations, fostering understanding and empathy. For example, youngsters undertaking their Duke of Edinburgh Awards can use this technology to share their skills, learn from people in care settings, and participate in collaborative projects. Let's consider a successful case where local school students used the Tiny Tablet to create digital storybooks based on residents' memories.

This activity not only offered students a unique perspective on history but also provided people in that care setting with a cherished memento and the pleasure of shared storytelling.

Chapter 22: Integrating Technology in Care Collaboration

Religious and Spiritual Engagement

The Tiny Tablet also makes it possible to live-stream religious services, ensuring that people can stay connected with their faith communities. Apart from watching services, people can use the tablet for spiritual reflection, prayer groups, and discussions. In one care home, residents used the Tiny Tablet to participate in a local church's virtual Bible study group, offering a sense of continuity and community during isolating times.

Collaborating with Local Groups and Organisations

The Tiny Tablet can facilitate digital partnerships with local charities, clubs, and businesses, enabling people to continue pursuing their interests and hobbies. In a birdwatching group, for example, people used the Tiny Tablet to participate in live birdwatching sessions, share observations, and discuss their findings with community members.

Building Community Events and Activities

The Tiny Tablet opens up new possibilities for organising virtual community events. From holiday celebrations to local traditions, individuals can be active participants in the community life. For instance, one care home organised a virtual community fair, where residents used the Tiny Tablet to "visit" stalls, interact with vendors, and even enjoy live performances.

Chapter 22: Integrating Technology in Care Collaboration

Boosting Communication with the Community

The Tiny Tablet can also amplify care settings' communication with the wider community. Social media platforms, websites, and digital newsletters can all be managed via the tablet, providing regular updates, sharing success stories, and crowdsourcing ideas or feedback from the community.

The Benefits and Impact of Community Engagement

The benefits of integrating the local community into care settings through technology are numerous. People experience improved mental, emotional, and social well-being. Success can be evaluated through the richness of relationships formed, the variety of activities engaged in, and the overall satisfaction of people with their community interactions.

Conclusion

Technology has the potential to revolutionise community involvement in care settings. A tool like the Tiny Tablet, which offers versatility and accessibility, can facilitate and enhance community connections. As we move forward, encouraging further community engagement through such technology is not only beneficial but essential in creating vibrant, fulfilling environments for residents in care.

Part VI: Navigating Challenges

Chapter 23: Managing Behaviour of Concern

Navigating behaviour of concern in care settings can indeed be a complex task. The challenge often becomes more pronounced when working with people living with conditions such as dementia or other cognitive impairments.

The key lies in embracing approaches that can stimulate the mind, body, and emotions, reducing instances of behavioural challenges.

Technology has risen to this occasion, presenting us with unique, engaging, and effective solutions.

Harnessing the Power of Tiny Tablets

The Tiny Tablets have emerged as a versatile tool in managing behaviours of concern. The design of these tablets allows quick switching between activities, thus maintaining the persons interest and mitigating feelings of distress. They are an excellent option for people who prefer solitude or aren't as enthusiastic about traditional activities in care.

Through an extensive range of apps, from games and drawing applications to musical platforms, caregivers can effectively engage people you support.

The versatility of the Tiny Tablet enables them to distract and immerse individuals in enjoyable activities, significantly reducing the chances of behavioural concerns surfacing.

Chapter 23: Managing Behaviour of Concern

A Structured Routine for Comprehensive Stimulation

The key to preventing behavioural issues is not just distraction, but prevention. Having a structured routine filled with cognitive, physical, and emotional stimulation activities is an effective strategy to keep people you support stimulated and engaged.

Exercise holds a significant spot in this routine. A variety of exercises, from breathing exercises to full-body workouts, can be easily facilitated through the Tiny Tablet. These activities are not only good for physical well-being but also release mood-boosting hormones like dopamine and serotonin.

Creative engagements, such as drawing, puzzles, or virtual gardening, also play an essential role in managing behaviours of concern. These activities trigger the release of reward chemicals in the brain, which can lead to a reduction in challenging behaviour and an increase in overall well-being.

Chapter 23: Managing Behaviour of Concern

Travel Back in Time and Build Connections

Reminiscence activities, such as touring familiar places on Google Earth or listening to favourite songs from the past, are highly beneficial. They offer both emotional and cognitive benefits to residents at all stages of dementia.

In addition to this, the Tiny Tablet serves as a bridge for social interactions. Through group video calls or other virtual interactions, People can stay connected with loved ones, adding an essential layer to their emotional well-being. Music therapy, facilitated through platforms like YouTube, provides visual and auditory stimulation and promotes the release of endorphins.

To sum it up, Tiny Tablets have revolutionised the approach to managing behaviour of concern. These innovative devices help reduce reliance on pharmaceutical interventions by engaging people you support in stimulating and enjoyable activities throughout the day.

By focusing on cognitive, physical, and emotional engagement, individuals stay active, stimulated, and satisfied, resulting in improved overall well-being.

This use of technology creates a happier, more serene living environment, thereby transforming the care experience for the people you support.

It's the dawn of a new era in care settings, and it's nothing short of remarkable!

Chapter 24: Release Happy Hormones Using Technology

Harnessing the power of technology can be a creative and effective way to positively influence the emotional state of the people you support.

By releasing the body's "happy hormones," technology-based activities can bring about a wide range of health benefits, including improving cognitive ability, boosting self-esteem, and managing stress and pain.

This chapter explores how technology, specifically touchscreen tables, can stimulate the production of these hormones, thereby enhancing the well-being of the people you support.

Understanding Happy Hormones

Dopamine

Often referred to as the "feel good" hormone, dopamine plays a significant role in your brain's reward system. It is associated with pleasurable sensations and is vital to learning, memory, and motor system function.

Serotonin

This hormone helps regulate mood, sleep, appetite, digestion, learning ability, and memory. An optimal level of serotonin contributes to a feeling of well-being and happiness.

Oxytocin

Known as the "love" hormone, oxytocin promotes trust, empathy, and bonding. Its levels usually increase with physical affection and human contact.

Endorphins

The body's natural pain reliever, endorphins are produced in response to stress or discomfort. Their levels also increase during rewarding activities like eating, exercise, challenges, and intimacy.

Chapter 24: Release Happy Hormones Using Technology

Harnessing Technology to Increase Happy Hormones

Touchscreen tables can be an incredible tool to stimulate the production of these hormones, enhancing the overall well-being of people you support.

Dopamine & Serotonin Boosting Activities

Activities like a daily exercise routine, listening to music, singing & dancing can stimulate dopamine and serotonin production. Coupled with a balanced diet, quality sleep, and light therapy, they can effectively boost these hormones.

Oxytocin Boosting Activities

Through listening or making music, reminiscing, physical contact, and social activities, oxytocin levels can be increased. Communication with loved ones, fussing dogs, breathing exercises, and sensory activities using lights and sounds are also effective.

Endorphin Boosting Activities

Fun and laughter, story times, music therapy, calming sensory time, meditation, competitive games, and arts and crafts can all help stimulate endorphin production.

Chapter 24: Release Happy Hormones Using Technology

Implementing Happy Hormone Boosting Activities

The touchscreen table is your one-stop tool to hack the happy hormones of the people you support. Here's how:

- **Music, Dance, and Exercise:** Use YouTube or apps like Spotify for music therapy sessions. Incorporate dance and exercise routines as well to get your people moving.
- **Reminiscence:** Utilise Google Earth for virtual tours to their favourite places or homes where they grew up, stimulating memories and conversations.
- **Breathing Exercises and Meditation:** Use dedicated apps or YouTube guides for these calming activities.
- **Arts & Crafts:** Painting by numbers, memory games, and more can be done using relevant apps.
- **Story Time:** Audio books are readily available and can be played directly from the table.
- **Contacting Loved Ones:** Keep those you support connected to their family and friends around the world using video calling apps like Zoom and Skype.
- **Cognitive Challenges:** Cognitive games stimulate the mind and can be found in abundance in the app store.
- **Sensory Fun:** Apps like Magic Fluids & Bubble Bliss offer colourful, interactive experiences that stimulate the senses.
- **Making Music:** Using apps like Perfect Piano/Drum Kit, individuals can enjoy creating music.
- **Competitions and Theme Nights:** Organise competitions and theme nights, creating a fun and interactive environment for the people you support.

Chapter 25: Addressing Staff Apprehension Towards Change

In every care environment, change is inevitable and necessary for progress. Yet, it is common to encounter apprehension and resistance among staff when new initiatives, particularly those involving technology, are introduced. We will will delve into why such apprehension occurs and present strategies to address it effectively.

Staff apprehension towards change can be attributed to a myriad of factors. These could range from concerns about increased workload, to a simple fear of the unknown.

It's crucial to empathise with these feelings, as dismissing them could lead to disengagement or resistance.

The Psychology of Change Resistance

Humans are creatures of habit, and the introduction of unfamiliar elements can trigger anxiety. Uncertainty about the potential impact of change can lead to fear and resistance.

Staff members might worry that new processes or technologies could add to their already demanding workload. It is critical to assure them that these changes are designed to make their jobs easier, not harder.

Another common concern is whether their current skills will suffice in a changing environment. This is particularly true when technology is involved.

Chapter 25: Addressing Staff Apprehension Towards Change

Strategies for Managing Change

Transparent communication is key. Ensure all staff members understand the reasons behind the change, the benefits it will bring, and the support available to them throughout the transition.

Involve staff in decision-making processes. When people feel their input is valued, they are more likely to support the change.

Overcoming Technological Hesitation

Many people are intimidated by technology, fearing they will make mistakes or not be able to learn how to use it. Address these fears with patience, understanding, and comprehensive training.

Proper training is crucial to build confidence and competence. Regular workshops and hands-on sessions can help staff members familiarise themselves with new technology.

The Role of Leadership in Change Management

Leaders should foster an environment where staff members feel comfortable voicing their concerns. Open dialogue can address fears, clarify misconceptions, and build consensus.

Leaders should embrace change and demonstrate its benefits. This positive attitude can trickle down and influence the entire team.

Chapter 25: Addressing Staff Apprehension Towards Change

Promoting the Benefits of Change

Focus on how these changes will improve care quality and individual experience. This positive outlook can motivate staff to embrace change.

Showcase how the new processes or technologies can streamline tasks, improve efficiency, and enable staff to dedicate more time to people they support.

Handling Resistance to Change

A phased approach can reduce resistance to change. This allows staff to adjust gradually and feel less overwhelmed.

Ensure staff members know that they have the support they need during the transition. Encourage team members to help each other and share their learning experiences.

The Path Forward

Embracing change can seem daunting, but it is a crucial part of improving care. By understanding staff apprehension, fostering open communication, providing adequate training, and demonstrating the benefits of change, leaders can ease the transition and make way for improved care quality and efficiency. Change, after all, is the path forward for better care.

Part VII: A Guide to Recommended Resources

Chapter 26: Exploring Additional Peripherals

Incorporating technology in care environments not only involves the primary devices such as tablets or touch screen activity tables but also includes a range of additional peripherals that can significantly enhance user experience and engagement.

These accessories can augment the existing functions and features, offering a more personalised and convenient way to enjoy technology. Let's delve into some of these peripherals and their benefits.

Easy-Grip Stylus Pens

A stylus pen is a useful tool that provides better control and precision when interacting with touch screen devices. However, for older people, especially those with mobility issues in their hands, using a regular stylus pen may be challenging. This is where easy-grip stylus pens come into play.

With a larger grip area, these pens are designed to be more comfortable and easier to handle, making them ideal for people who may struggle with finer motor skills. The easier grip can help them engage more fully with drawing apps, writing activities, and games that require precise touch, thereby enhancing their overall experience.

Chapter 26: Exploring Additional Peripherals

Bluetooth Headphones

With Bluetooth headphones, people can enjoy their favourite music, movies, or interactive games without disturbing others. They provide a more personalised experience and enable people to fully immerse themselves in the digital activities they love.

In addition, these headphones can be a great tool for people with hearing difficulties. They can adjust the volume to their comfort level, ensuring they don't miss out on any part of the audio content.

Pedal Exercisers for Virtual Cycle Tours

Exercise is essential for the those in care, contributing to both physical and mental health. With pedal exercisers, individuals can embark on virtual cycling tours while staying active and engaged.

Using Google Earth or other VR apps in conjunction with pedal exercisers, individuals can explore various locations around the globe, making their workout sessions more fun and engaging.

From cycling along scenic coastal paths to navigating through bustling city streets, virtual cycle tours can turn exercise into an exciting adventure.

Chapter 26: Exploring Additional Peripherals

HDMI Sound Bars

Sound plays a crucial role in the overall media consumption experience. Whether it's listening to golden oldies, watching a favourite movie, or playing a memory game with audio cues, having clear and high-quality sound can significantly enhance the experience.

HDMI sound bars connected to your touchscreen table can provide superior audio performance. They can make the music come alive, provide clearer dialogues in movies, and enhance the overall auditory feedback from games or apps. They're especially beneficial when organising group activities or theme nights, filling the room with immersive sound.

Additional peripherals not only provide enhanced user experiences but also cater to individual needs and preferences of the people you support.

By integrating these accessories with your core technology, you can ensure that all those you support, regardless of their physical abilities or personal preferences, can reap the benefits of digital engagement, thus enriching their overall quality of life.

Chapter 27: Navigating the Play Store App Guide

The following list of free to download apps has been is accurate as of April 2023, all available to download from the Google Play Store and enjoy with the people you support.

Chapter 27: Navigating the Play Store App Guide

Silhouette Art

Doodle Art

Art Puzzle

Knitting Genius

Koto Connect

All Musical Instruments

Flower Arrangement

Imaginarie

Sketch a Day

Loop

Wood Blocks

Bricks Breaker

Free Jigsaw

Maze Path of Light

Suduko

Candy Crush

Pictawords

Cross Words

Word Brain

Maths Duel

Kahoot

World History Quiz

Wheel of Fortune

Water Sort

Word search by Wixot

Words with Friends

Mahjong

Flow Water Fountain

Puzzledom

Chapter 27: Navigating the Play Store App Guide

Mind Mate

Acuity Games

My House of Memories

Alzheimers Cards

Neuro Nation

InspireD

Recover Brain

MyLifeTV

Numendoom Memory training

Mind Pal

Train Your Brain Visuospatial

Train Your Brain Memory

Train Your Brain Coordination

Train Your Brain Attention

Train Your Brain Reasoning

Train Your Brain Language

Train Your brain Senior Games

Pastimes 14 in 1 S

ensory Fish

Pop Us!

Harmony

Galaxy Particles Sensory Plasma

Night Light

Medito

Mesmerize

Orbia

Magic Flames

Silk Paints

Calm

Chapter 27: Navigating the Play Store App Guide

Drawing Desk

Coloring Book for Adults

Cake Coloring 3d

Lets Create Pottery Perfect Piano

Knitting Master

Drum Kit

Colorfy

Marimba Xylophone

Focus - Train your Brain Carnival Games

2 Player Pastimes

Brain Games

Imaglze

Gin Rummy

Senior Fitness

Guess That Song Bowling Club

Darts King

General Knowledge Quiz

Who Wants to be a Millionaire

4 in a Row

Chess

Checkers

Bridge

Air Hockey Challenge

Terrarium

Golf Nest

8 Ball Pool

Scrabble

Monopoly

Bingo

Chapter 27: Navigating the Play Store App Guide

Zen Pinball

Space Invaders

3d Tennis

Fishing Life

Pacman

Train Station

Flight Pilot Simulator

Badminton League

Trivial Pursuit

Block Puzzle

Golf Strike

Rummikub

Word Wow Around the World

World Basket Ball King

Archery Battle

Brain Games

Puzzle Hub

General Knowledge Quiz Brain Plus

Hearts Card Game

Word Logic - Trivia Puzzles Yahtzy

Water Sort

Jeopardy

Riddle me

Cricket League

Mini Golf

Ping Pong Fury

Hidden journey Objects Puzzle

Kettlemind Competitive Brain

Mini Football

Chapter 27: Navigating the Play Store App Guide

Wikipedia

YouTube

Google Earth

Google Drive

Zoom

Skype

Gmail

Google Chrome

Dominoes

Roulette Royale Solitaire

Zynga Poker

Angry Birds

Shine

Panic Attack Anxiety Relief

Looper

Art Puzzle

Magic Cross Stitch

Magic Colour

Finger Painting

Cross Stitch by Numbers

Fireworks Colour

Real Guitar

Sketchbook

Doodle Master

Harp Real

Roll The Ball

Flow Free

Smart Puzzles Collection

Tetris

Chapter 27: Navigating the Play Store App Guide

Math

Jeopardy

Trivia 360

Famous People History Quiz

Quiz: Logo Game

Flower Memory Game

A Better Visit

Flower Garden

1 Player Pastimes

Audible

Tunein

Google Duo

Google Docs

Google Translate

Google News

Weather App

Spotify

Vimeo

BBC News

BBC Sport

BBC Weather

Magic Fluids

Baby Bubbles

My Reef 3d

Light Box

Water Garden Fireworks

Anti Stress

Relax Melodies

Nature Sounds Relaxing Sounds

Conclusion

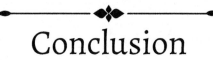

Conclusion

As we reach the conclusion of our enlightening journey, it's time to take a moment and reflect on the transformational power technology holds for the world of care. From video calls to virtual tours, from mind-stimulating games to sensory apps, we've explored an exciting range of digital tools, each contributing to the enhanced wellbeing of our residents.

We started our journey by highlighting the importance of technology in care settings, underscoring its ability to bridge gaps, connect people, and stimulate minds. Through 'Virtual Visits,' we saw how technology shrinks physical distances, enabling people to maintain personal connections with their loved ones and healthcare providers.

Meanwhile, we emphasised the power of virtual exploration and reminiscence, broadening horizons and sparking enriching conversations among those in care.

We demonstrated how easy and accessible language learning can be with YouTube tutorials. We also delved into the joy of endless information discovery via Wikipedia and the immense potential that Google Chrome holds for enriching the browsing experience.

Emphasising the cognitive stimulation possibilities, we highlighted the role of brain games, puzzle games, and other interactive apps in engaging and challenging people, encouraging social interaction and friendly competition.

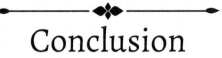

Conclusion

Focusing on creativity, we appreciated the opportunities provided by arts and crafts apps, allowing people you support to express their artistic inclinations. We also recognised the importance of sensory stimulation, showcasing sensory apps' ability to reduce anxiety, improve mood, and promote social interaction, a crucial aspect of healthy aging.

Chapter 21 introduced the "My Story So Far" fact-finding approach, underlining the importance of tracking and documenting progress to personalise well-being care. We then addressed behavioural concerns and explored strategies to manage them, acknowledging the substantial positive impact technology can have on a persons behaviour.

In subsequent chapters, we dealt with staff apprehension and fears, proposing strategies for change management. This was followed by a deep dive into the power of harnessing 'Happy Hormones' using technology, a crucial element for a persons well-being.

Further, we introduced a variety of additional peripherals, demonstrating how they can enhance the user experience and cater to individual needs. And finally, we navigated the impressive world of Google Play Store, presenting a comprehensive guide to some of the most impactful apps in healthcare.

Technology, as we've discovered, is not only a tool but a companion in the journey of care and support. Its power to engage, entertain, stimulate, and connect is undeniably transformative. It is our hope that the insights offered in this book will inspire you to embrace and harness this power to its fullest potential.

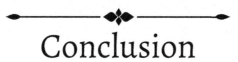

Conclusion

As we move forward, let's remember that at the heart of it all is the human connection, the warmth, and the care we extend to the people we support

While technology offers us fantastic tools to enhance this, it is our empathy, compassion, and dedication that make the real difference.

Thank you for joining us on this journey. We trust that the knowledge and strategies shared will empower you to create an even more engaging, vibrant, and stimulating environment for the people you support.

Here's to embracing change, welcoming innovation, and shaping a brighter, happier future for care!

For further information or advice, please visit us at www.inspired-inspirations.com